R.S. PATRICK
Liver Pathology

OXFORD COLOUR ATLASES OF PATHOLOGY

1. LIVER PATHOLOGY by R.S. Patrick

In preparation
   PEDIATRIC PATHOLOGY by H. Cameron
   SKIN PATHOLOGY by W.A.J. Crane
   NEUROPATHOLOGY by R.O. Weller
   GYNECOLOGICAL PATHOLOGY by W.B. Robertson
   CARDIOVASCULAR PATHOLOGY by M.J. Davies
   GASTROINTESTINAL PATHOLOGY by B.C. Morson
   HEMATOLOGY by J.E. MacIver
   LYMPHOID TISSUE PATHOLOGY by D.H. Wright
   OBSTETRIC & PERINATAL PATHOLOGY by D.I. Rushton
   RENAL PATHOLOGY by J.R. Tighe
   ENDOCRINE PATHOLOGY by A. Munro Neville

OXFORD COLOUR ATLASES OF PATHOLOGY
GENERAL EDITOR: R.C. CURRAN, MD·FRCP·FRS(Edinburgh)·FRC Path

COLOUR ATLAS OF
Liver
Pathology

BY R.S. PATRICK, MD·FRC Path

WITH 432 ILLUSTRATIONS IN COLOUR

HARVEY MILLER PUBLISHERS
OXFORD UNIVERSITY PRESS

Originating Publisher HARVEY MILLER LTD
20 Marryat Road·London SW19 5BD·England

Published in conjunction with OXFORD UNIVERSITY PRESS
Walton Street·Oxford OX2 6DP

Oxford·London·Glasgow
New York·Toronto·Melbourne·Wellington
Kuala Lumpur·Singapore·Hong Kong·Tokyo
Delhi·Bombay·Calcutta·Madras·Karachi
Nairobi·Dar es Salaam·Cape Town

Published in the United States by
OXFORD UNIVERSITY PRESS·NEW YORK

British Library Cataloguing in Publication Data
Patrick, R.S.
    Colour atlas of liver pathology.——
    (Oxford colour atlases of pathology)
    1. Liver —— Diseases
    I. Title
    616.3′6207   RC847

ISBN 0-19-921033-0

MADE IN SWITZERLAND
Illustrations originated by Schwitter AG·Basle
Printed and bound by Arts Graphiques Coop Suisse·Basle
Text set by Advanced Filmsetters (Glasgow) Ltd·Glasgow·Scotland

Contents

Editor's Foreword

'A picture shows me at a glance what it takes dozens of pages of a book to expound.' (Turgenev: FATHERS AND SONS, ch. 16).

HISTOPATHOLOGY IS CONCERNED with the derangements of tissue structure that occur in disease, traditionally as revealed by the study of stained histological sections with the light microscope. It has long been realised that the structure of the tissues (microscopic and macroscopic), their function, and their chemical composition are intimately and inextricably linked; and that in disease all three are almost certain to be altered. It is only in recent years however that it has proved possible to demonstrate this effectively, as a result of the revolution which histopathology has undergone, and which has turned it into one of the most rapidly-advancing branches of medical science, with a rate and type of development suggesting that its potential is almost unlimited.

The revolution in histopathology has been based both on developments within the subject itself and also through its interaction with other clinical and scientific disciplines. Thus microscopy has advanced remarkably, culminating in various forms of electron microscopy. The methods used for identifying the chemical components of the tissues have also improved steadily; and immuno-histochemical techniques of great sensitivity, often using monoclonal antibodies of absolute specificity, are becoming available at an increasing rate. At the same time as these technical improvements have been occurring, the range of tissues and specimens available to the pathologist has increased dramatically, with the increasing application of the clinical techniques of needle biopsy and endoscopy. The repeated sampling of diseased tissues which these techniques allow has made it possible for the first time to obtain a 'moving picture' of the evolution of many disease processes in man; and the functional and prognostic significance of the 'still' picture of the structural changes detectable by light microscopy in ordinary histological preparations obtainable from a single specimen or biopsy can now be assessed with precision and confidence. Concurrently clinical practice has become increasingly specialised with the formation of highly expert groups, often concerned with a single body system, in which the histopathologist generally plays a highly significant and often central role.

While it is accepted that there is no adequate substitute for experience in handling and studying tissues from surgical operations and necropsies, the increase in breadth and depth of histopathology has been so great that no pathologist, however extensive his routine experience, can keep abreast of all the developments in the subject; and must soon find that his knowledge is inadequate.

The Oxford Atlases, of which the present volume is the first to be published, are intended to help the practising pathologist to remedy this, by adding to the body of knowledge on which he depends. They should make it possible for him to become familiar with and to recognise a much wider range of lesions than he would otherwise encounter, and to interpret and solve more effectively the problems which he encounters in his daily practice.

Professor Patrick's book is based on many years' practical experience of liver disease, in this and other countries, and particularly Africa.

The illustrations are of the highest quality. Most are of common conditions but uncommon and rare conditions are included for completeness. Great care has been taken in the preparation and selection of specimens, and the macroscopic illustrations are wherever possible of unfixed tissues in order to match the appearances of those encountered at operation or necropsy. The large majority of the microscopic preparations are histological; and a feature of the book is the considerable number of low-power photomicrographs giving comprehensive views of a variety of lesions. Considerable care has been taken in the reproduction of these, to preserve the fine detail present in them. Special staining techniques are illustrated where they contribute significantly, and newer techniques of proven value including a number of immunohistochemical preparations are included. Professor Patrick's extensive experience in experimental pathology is readily detectable, but his Atlas is essentially a clinico-pathological treatise aimed at the practising postgraduate pathologist and at clinicians with an interest in liver disease.

It is hoped that this book and all subsequent volumes in the Oxford series will provide vivid and memorable images, at all levels from the macroscopic to the molecular, of the derangements of structure which underlie the malfunctioning of tissues and organs which manifest themselves clinically as disease. The Oxford Atlases are not textbooks, but are intended to complement the standard textbooks. The text is therefore concise but nevertheless always includes a full description of each of the lesions illustrated as well as relevant information regarding its pathogenesis and functional and clinical significance.

R. C. Curran, 1982

Preface

THE REMARKABLE EXPANSION of knowledge of human pathology during the past few decades now makes it very difficult for any one hospital pathologist to provide the level of advice required by many of his clinical colleagues in various medical and surgical specialities. This is particularly true of hepatology where the interpretation of biopsy material is so often essential to the diagnosis and management of cases of liver disease. There is no substitute for personal experience in gaining proficiency in this work, but this must be based on a sound knowledge of liver histopathology. It is the purpose of this Atlas to assist in laying such a foundation by illustrating typical gross and light-microscopic appearances of liver disease which may be encountered by the clinical pathologist.

The Atlas consists of prints taken from colour transparencies which illustrate a wide range of disorders. Inessential repetition has been avoided but a few important conditions are shown in more than one chapter where this has been necessary to provide a comprehensive account of main topics. Some examples of experimental liver injury are included where these may help to clarify an understanding of comparable human conditions.

Many of the captions include comments on the main features of the disease which are illustrated. These are rather brief as the book is intended to supplement rather than to replace standard works on liver pathology. A short bibliography of such works is included.

The illustrations have been carefully selected mainly from a large number of specimens collected over many years by the author alone. It would be impossible to find a good example of every known condition in such a collection, and the assistance of many colleagues who have supplied valuable material is gratefully acknowledged. These are: Dr. R. A. Burnett, Department of Pathology, Stobhill General Hospital, Glasgow (*9.32, 9.33, 11.13*); Dr. David Doyle, Department of Neuropathology, Southern General Hospital, Glasgow (*12.15*); Dr. A. A. M. Gibson, Department of Pathology, Royal Hospital for Sick Children, Glasgow (*9.19*); Dr. F. D. Lee, Department of Pathology, Royal Infirmary, Glasgow (*3.31, 3.32, 5.35, 6.29, 8.20, 8.21, 8.22, 10.64, 10.65*); Dr. G. A. McDonald, Department of Hematology, Royal Infirmary, Glasgow (*12.11, 12.12, 12.13, 12.14*); Professor J. O'D. McGee, Department of Pathology, University of Oxford (*3.36, 5.14, 7.24, 9.37, 9.38, 9.41, 10.60*); Dr. R. I. Russell, Department of Gastroenterology, Royal Infirmary, Glasgow (*12.8*); Dr. W. G. S. Spilg, Department of Pathology, Victoria Infirmary, Glasgow (*10.32, 10.33, 10.34*); Dr. Than Than, Department of Pathology, Institute of Medicine, Mandalay (*8.23, 8.24*).

All illustrations have been prepared from photographs taken by the author. In this task much encouragement and helpful advice have been received from the editor of this series, Professor R. C. Curran, particularly with respect to colour correction and definition of low-power photomicrographs. This most valuable assistance is gratefully acknowledged. Thanks are due to Mrs. M. Thomson and Mrs. I. Main, Department of Pathology, Glasgow Royal Infirmary, for secretarial assistance. It is a pleasure also to acknowledge the co-operation and guidance of Harvey and Elly Miller in the preparation of this book.

CHAPTER 1

Normal Liver

1.1 Normal liver: anterior surface

The large right lobe and much smaller left lobe are separated by a thin fibrous band which is the attachment of the falciform ligament to the anterior surface of the liver. This ligament consists of two closely applied layers of peritoneum connecting liver to the undersurface of the diaphragm and anterior abdominal wall. The tip of the gall bladder protrudes below the inferior margin of the right lobe.

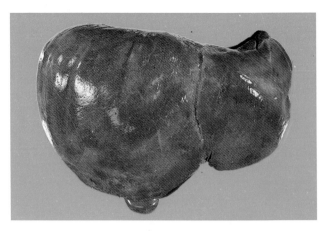

1.1 Normal liver: anterior surface.

1.2 Normal liver: inferior surface

Parts of both right and left lobes are seen. The upper part of the right lobe is devoid of a peritoneal covering ('bare area' of liver). It has a groove containing the inferior vena cava which is laid open and shows two hepatic venous ostia at its upper end. The small caudate lobe is the portion of the liver immediately to the left of the vena cava and is separated from the left lobe by the deep fissure for the ligamentum venosum. Inferiorly, the gall bladder to the right and the fissure for the ligamentum teres to the left are separated by the small quadrate lobe. Above this lobe in the centre of the field is the porta hepatis where hepatic artery, portal vein, lymphatic vessels, nerves and bile ducts enter or emerge.

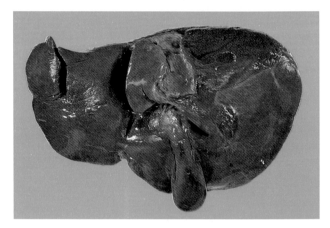

1.2 Normal liver: inferior surface.

1.3 Normal liver: cut surface

This shows the uniform reddish-brown colour of the organ. It is possible to detect its constituent lobules, each about 1 mm in diameter. These are more distinct in many diffuse pathological conditions, e.g. **4.16**. Several transected portal and intrahepatic veins are seen readily.

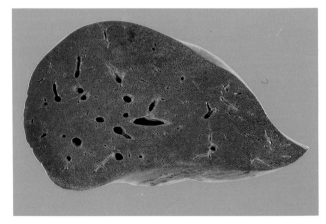

1.3 Normal liver: cut surface.

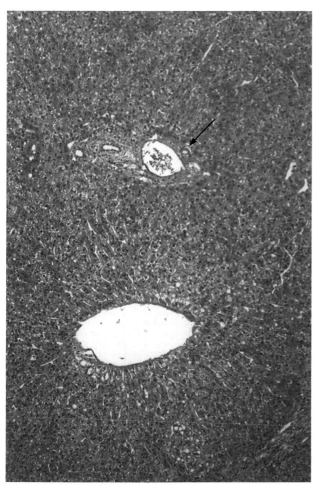

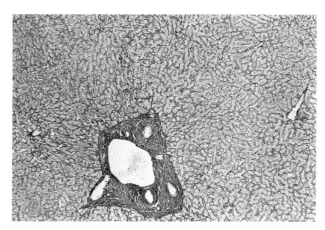

1.5 Normal liver.

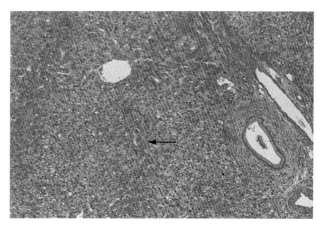

1.4 Normal liver.

1.6 Normal liver.

1.4 Normal liver

The portal tract (above) contains a dilated portal vein to the right of which is a small hepatic arteriole (arrow). On its left is a small interlobular bile duct lined by cuboidal epithelium. A few tiny bile ductular channels with similar lining are present here and in part of a second portal tract (bottom right). Between these tracts there is a prominent dilated centrilobular vein. The hepatocytes are arranged in plates separated by narrow or collapsed sinusoidal channels. × 88 Hematoxylin and eosin.

1.5 Normal liver

The normal trabecular pattern is prominent in sections stained for reticulin, which outlines the walls of sinusoids. Plates of hepatocytes in the normal adult are mostly one cell thick. There is a portal tract (lower centre) and a small centrilobular venule (centre right). × 75 Reticulin stain.

1.6 Normal liver

A fibrous septum crosses the field diagonally from above and to the right. It contains a prominent septal bile duct cut transversely; this has a muscle coat and lining of columnar epithelium. Beside it is a portal vein with elongated lumen. Above these vessels there is an interlobular bile duct cut longitudinally with a lining of cuboidal epithelium. A centrilobular vein is present on the left of the field, and in the centre is a tiny bile ductule—Canal of Hering (arrow). × 75 Hematoxylin and eosin.

1.7 Normal mouse liver: cytoplasmic granules

At high magnification rather coarse basophilic granules are seen in hepatocyte cytoplasm. The granules represent arrays of rough endoplasmic reticulum and are an index of normal protein synthesis. They disappear quickly when these organelles are damaged by any means (**4.2**). They are less conspicuous in light microscopic preparations of human liver. × 300 Hematoxylin and eosin.

1.8 Normal liver: glycogen content

Periodic acid-Schiff staining of paraffin sections shows purple glycogen in the cytoplasm of many hepatocytes throughout the liver lobule. Staining is negative after pretreatment of the section with diastase. Glycogen disappears quickly after death or when there has been delay in fixation. It diminishes also with fasting and smaller amounts tend to be confined within centrilobular hepatocytes. × 117 Periodic acid-Schiff and hematoxylin.

1.9 Mitotic activity

Mitotic activity may be seen during recovery from various types of liver damage, and three hepatocytes in this field contain mitotic figures (small arrows). The remaining normal hepatocytes have typical round nuclei, prominent nucleoli and substantial cytoplasm. A number of smaller sinusoidal lining cells are present, one of which is indicated by a large arrow; they also can show mitotic activity in regenerating liver. × 300 Hematoxylin and eosin.

1.10 Fetal liver

A sixteen-week fetal liver in which hepatocytes are arranged in trabeculae which are several cells thick. Part of a large portal tract (right) contains rather loose areolar connective tissue. During ante-natal life the liver is an important site for blood formation; the illustration shows numerous nucleated blood cells in sinusoids and to a lesser extent in portal tract connective tissue. × 88 Hematoxylin and eosin.

1.11 Fetal liver

Reticulin appears as very thin black lines which partly delineate the walls of many sinusoids. Therefore, this method of staining outlines the relatively thick trabeculae. The small round nuclei of numerous hematopoietic cells are more deeply counterstained with neutral red than those of the larger hepatocytes. × 187 Reticulin stain.

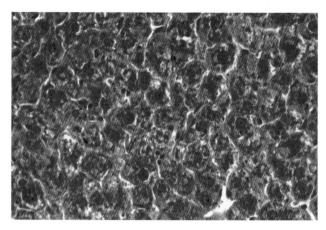

1.7 Normal mouse liver: cytoplasmic granules.

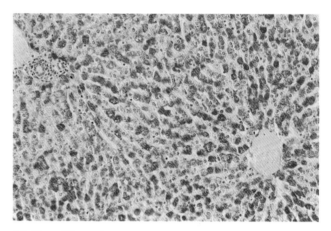

1.8 Normal liver: glycogen content.

1.12 Neonatal liver

The appearances are generally similar to embryonic liver but portal tract connective tissue, as seen on the upper left, is less conspicuous. Hematopoietic cells are still prominent but less numerous. × 117 Hematoxylin and eosin.

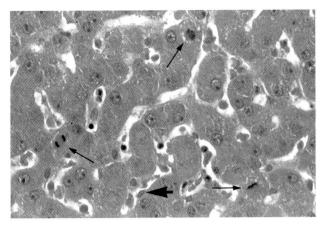

1.9 Mitotic activity.

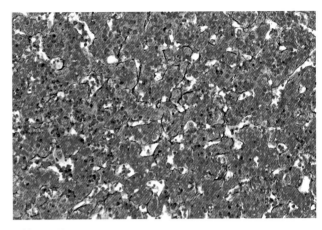

1.11 Fetal liver.

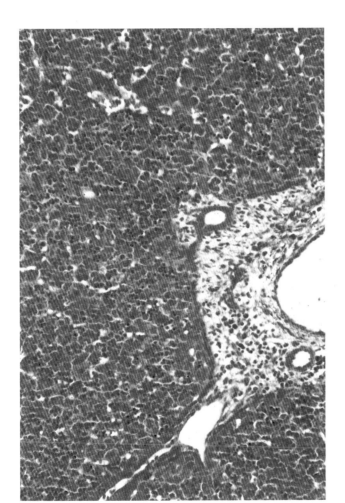

1.10 Fetal liver.

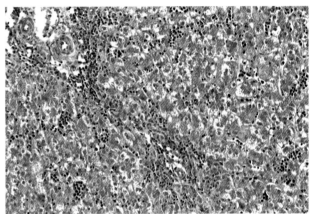

1.12 Neonatal liver.

1.13 Extramedullary hematopoiesis in adult liver

Following destruction of bone marrow by disease in adult life there can be reversion to blood cell formation in the liver and in other organs, such as spleen or renal pelvis. This liver is from a patient who suffered from fibrosis of bone marrow. There are many small nucleated blood cells in the sinusoids together with several megakaryocytes which are conspicuous because of their relatively large size and irregularly-shaped deeply-staining nuclei. × 187 Hematoxylin and eosin.

1.14 Extramedullary hematopoiesis in adult liver

Hematopoiesis may also occur in adult liver as a manifestation of recovery from bone marrow depression. This is a rather extreme case in a patient with alcoholic hepatitis. The biopsy was taken two days after the institution of treatment for severe folate deficiency; while it contains leucocytes which are part of the inflammatory reaction induced by alcohol, it also shows a prominent hematopoietic reaction with numerous nucleated red cells, myeloid cells and two megakaryocytes (arrows). × 117 Hematoxylin and eosin.

1.15 Lipochrome pigment

Many small granules of brown lipofuscin are present in hepatocyte cytoplasm, especially in cells near the centrilobular vein (above). A few Kupffer cells contain ceroid pigment which is periodic acid-Schiff (PAS)—positive (arrow). These are two types of lipochrome pigment: lipofuscin being seen frequently in the liver of elderly patients, of patients with some wasting disease and of patients following intake of phenacetin; and ceroid pigment, which indicates macrophage activity following various types of liver injury. × 187 Periodic acid-Schiff and hematoxylin after diastase.

1.16 Ceroid pigment

A prominent collection of macrophages which contains this purple-staining pigment. In unstained sections it has a dull brown or yellow colour. The material is derived by phagocytosis of lipid and other products of hepatocytic disintegration. In this case, liver damage was attributed to the administration of an excessive dose of tetracycline, a drug which is responsible also for the severe fatty change present in surviving hepatocytes. × 187 Periodic acid-Schiff and hematoxylin after diastase.

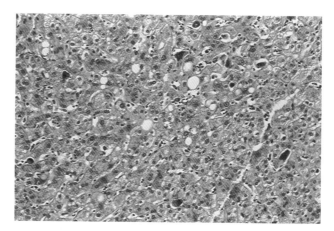

1.13 Extramedullary hematopoiesis in adult liver.

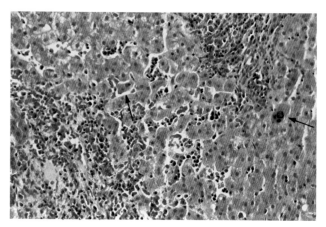

1.14 Extramedullary hematopoiesis in adult liver.

1.17 Normal infant liver: hemosiderin

The liver from a six-week infant showing much hemosiderin in hepatocytes and Kupffer cells. This pigment, which gives a positive Prussian blue reaction, appears within a week of birth and gradually disappears at about six to nine months of age. × 117 Perls' stain.

1.18 Normal liver: ageing

In elderly patients binucleate hepatocytes may be prominent, while other liver cells may be enlarged and have large hyperchromatic nuclei. These features should not be mistaken for unusual regenerative activity. They are present on the right of this field, the hepatocytes on the left being of normal morphology. × 187 Hematoxylin and eosin.

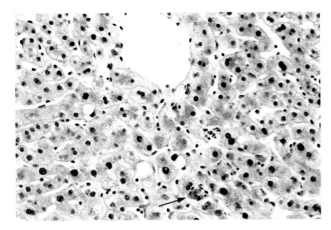

1.15 Lipochrome pigment.

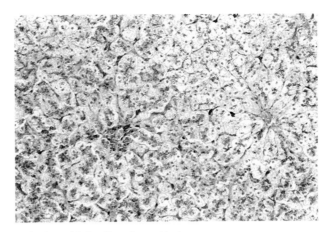

1.17 Normal infant liver: hemosiderin.

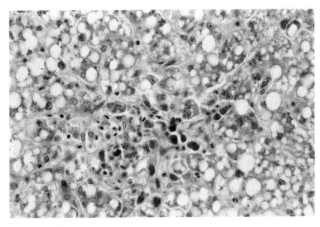

1.16 Ceroid pigment.

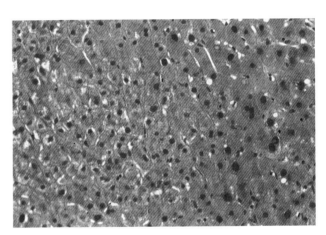

1.18 Normal liver: ageing.

1.19 Prominence of perisinusoidal cells

The vacuolated cells are perisinusoidal cells which lie in Disse's space. Electron microscopy of normal liver shows this space between hepatocytes and the thin cytoplasmic processes of sinusoidal lining cells. By light microscopy sinusoidal lining cells and perisinusoidal cells cannot be readily differentiated unless, as in this case, there is undue prominence of the normal fat storage function of the latter, since this gives rise to the vacuolated appearance. Ingestion of certain drugs, e.g. methotrexate or excessive amounts of Vitamin A can have this effect. Perisinusoidal cells are related also to the normal reticulin framework of the liver, another component of Disse's space, and are probably modified fibroblasts. When there is stimulation of hepatic fibrogenesis by induction of hepatic injury, perisinusoidal cells proliferate and appear to synthesize collagen. × 234 Hematoxylin and eosin.

1.20 Kupffer cell hyperactivity

Kupffer cells are members of the monocyte/macrophage category of cells and are situated on the lining of hepatic sinusoids. However, they are distinct from sinusoidal lining cells and from perisinusoidal cells. They are prominent in this field because of the exaggeration of their phagocytic activity and many have ingested red blood cells (arrow). The process of erythrophagocytosis was a manifestation of hemolytic anemia in this patient. × 353 Hematoxylin and eosin.

1.21 Fat-laden macrophages in portal tracts

The portal tract is expanded by numerous macrophages containing triglyceride. Unlike ceroid, the fat is unpigmented. It was derived by phagocytosis of focal collections of extracellular fat (fat cysts, **5.2**) and subsequent emigration of the macrophages to portal tracts. When there is a foreign body-type cell reaction in such lesions, the presence of mineral oil should be suspected (**4.47**). This can be derived from ingested liquid paraffin or from suppositories via the portal blood supply. × 117 Hematoxylin and eosin.

1.22 Subcapsular fibrosis

A thickened Glisson's capsule is seen above with fibrosis of underlying portal tracts. This latter feature becomes less prominent in deeper parts of the specimen (below). Care must be taken in assessing portal fibrosis from superficial biopsies. Moreover, zonal necrosis is often more severe and may even become confluent in subcapsular liver parenchyma (**4.18**). It is often desirable to undertake needle aspiration biopsy even during laparotomy in order to obtain a more accurate assessment of the severity of a diffuse lesion. × 28 Hematoxylin and eosin.

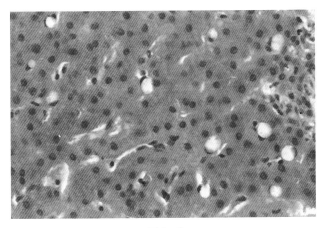

1.19 Prominence of perisinusoidal cells.

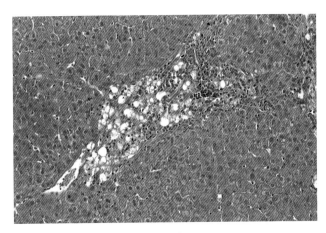

1.21 Fat-laden macrophages in portal tracts.

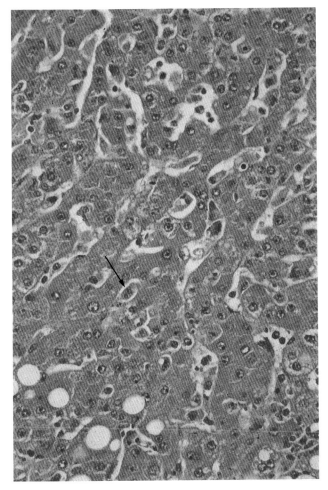

1.20 Kupffer cell hyperactivity.

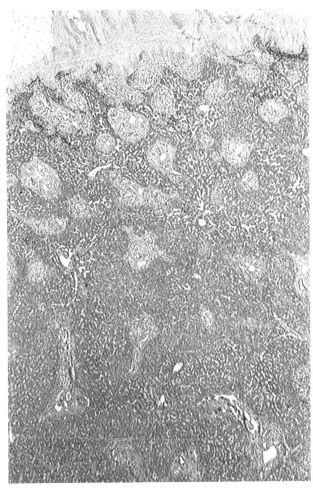

1.22 Subcapsular fibrosis.

CHAPTER 2

Cholestasis and Biliary Obstruction

2.1 Intrahepatic cholestasis

The presence of centrilobular bile pigment imparts a green mottled appearance to the liver surface. Green discoloration will be accentuated by formalin fixation. This patient had a fibrous stricture of the common bile duct without cholangitis.

2.2 Intrahepatic cholestasis: centrilobular

There are numerous small dark plugs of bile within distended bile capillaries. These are localized mostly to the central part of the liver lobule (left). In Van Gieson preparations, bile is usually dark olive green in colour as it is in tissue treated by chromate fixatives. In this section there is no other abnormality of note, and no indication of the cause of bile retention. It could indicate a disturbance of bile excretion in various types of hepatocyte damage (intrahepatic cholestasis) or be a consequence of large bile duct obstruction (extrahepatic cholestasis). × 75 Van Gieson's stain and hematoxylin.

2.3 Intrahepatic cholestasis: centrilobular

A higher magnification showing cholestasis round a centrilobular venule. Some hepatocytes are swollen, especially those adjacent to this vessel. Many contain small discrete granules of brown lipofuscin pigment. By contrast bile forms coarser dark green deposits mainly in distended bile capillaries and within macrophages. Hepatocyte damage including hydropic swelling, shrinkage and necrosis together with mild inflammatory changes should be regarded as a consequence and not a cause of the cholestasis, provided they are confined to the bile retention zones. Therefore, such appearances do not indicate the underlying cause of cholestasis. × 234 Van Gieson's stain and hematoxylin.

2.4 Intrahepatic cholestasis: periportal

Several dark bile plugs are seen in bile capillaries close to chronic portal inflammation (above). Unlike centrilobular cholestasis, this can be explained simply by obstruction to the onward flow of bile into fibrotic portal tracts where there is distortion or destruction of bile ductules. Accordingly, it may be found in cases of chronic portal and periportal inflammation from many causes but especially in primary biliary cirrhosis and in cholangiohepatitis secondary to large bile duct obstruction. × 134 Hematoxylin and eosin.

2.5 Chronic biliary disease: hyaline degeneration of hepatocytes

In chronic biliary disease, the periportal liver parenchyma often undergoes degenerative changes and destruction. In this case of primary biliary cirrhosis many hepatocytes adjacent to the inflamed portal tract above have disappeared while others show hydropic or hyaline degeneration. Two examples of the latter are indicated by arrows. Unlike alcoholic hepatitis, hyaline degeneration in biliary disease has this periportal distribution. × 187 Hematoxylin and eosin.

2.6 Chronic biliary disease: copper retention

Another feature of periportal hepatocytes in chronic biliary disease is copper retention which can be very prominent, especially in primary biliary cirrhosis. This section from such a case shows many small dark granules of copper-binding protein stained by orcein. × 146 Orcein.

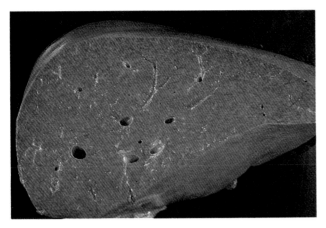

2.1 Intrahepatic cholestasis.

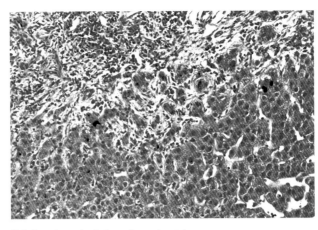

2.4 Intrahepatic cholestasis: periportal.

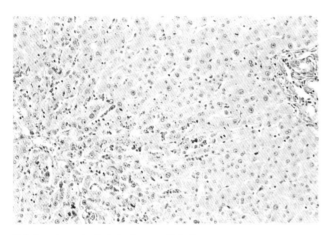

2.2 Intrahepatic cholestasis: centrilobular.

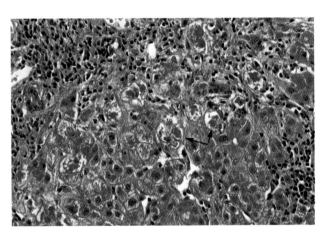

2.5 Chronic biliary disease: hyaline degeneration of hepatocytes.

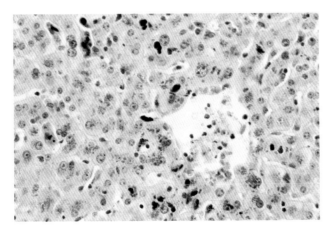

2.3 Intrahepatic cholestasis: centrilobular.

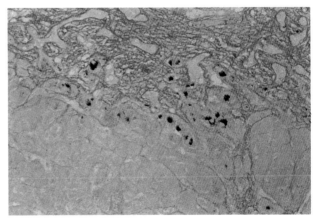

2.6 Chronic biliary disease: copper retention.

2.7 Bile pigment in Kupffer cells

In various types of liver damage, Kupffer cells become prominent through the ingestion of bile pigment, hemosiderin, and products of tissue disintegration which stain by the periodic acid-Schiff technique before or after diastase treatment. This purple staining of swollen Kupffer cells is evident here (large arrow). Plugs of bile in bile capillaries are brown in colour (small arrow). Prominent Kupffer cells may persist in the liver for several weeks after relief of obstructive jaundice. × 134 Periodic acid-Schiff and hematoxylin.

2.8 Intrahepatic cholestasis in hepatitis

This may be a feature of persistent hepatitis, including that due to drug-induced injury, viral infection and alcohol, when jaundice becomes mainly cholestatic in type. As in this biopsy from a patient with persistent viral hepatitis, bile plugs (arrows) have an irregular distribution in the lobule. Hepatocyte degenerative changes, especially hydropic swelling, are extensive, being attributable to the virus infection and are not, as in the case illustrated in **2.3**, confined to areas of cholestasis. × 113 Van Gieson's stain and hematoxylin.

2.9 Intrahepatic cholestasis in hepatitis

In this case chronic hepatitis was due to alcohol. The liver is very fatty and there is infiltration with inflammatory cells including neutrophil polymorphs (top left). Some hepatocytes have formed acinar structures each containing dark bile pigment. A similar arrangement of hepatocytes with or without cholestasis is seen in other forms of chronic hepatitis and probably represents regenerative activity (**7.4**). × 187 Hematoxylin and eosin.

2.10 Intrahepatic cholestasis in cirrhosis

This is an advanced case of cryptogenic cirrhosis, the liver parenchyma consisting of nodules separated by bands of fibrous connective tissue containing numbers of small bile ducts and ductules. Several of these channels are distended with inspissated dark brown bile pigment. This phenomenon is not confined to primary and secondary biliary cirrhosis and arises, presumably, from interference with bile flow in distorted bile channels occurring in cirrhosis of any type. In some cases of cirrhosis cholestasis involves bile capillaries (**6.10**) but it is absent in many others. × 71 Hematoxylin and eosin.

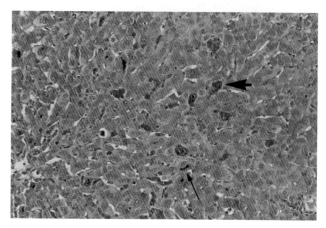

2.7 Bile pigment in Kupffer cells.

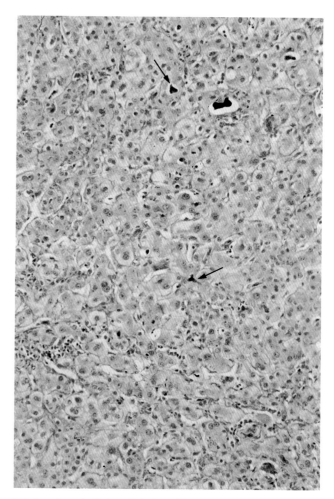

2.8 Intrahepatic cholestasis in hepatitis.

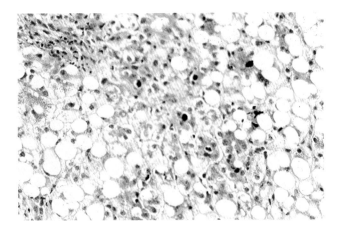

2.9 Intrahepatic cholestasis in hepatitis.

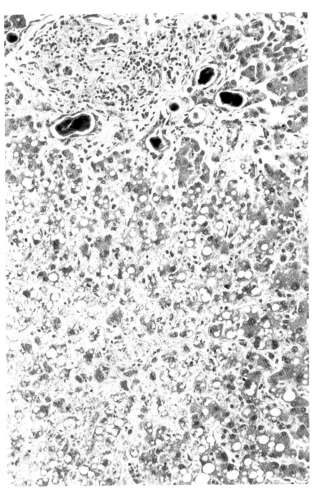

2.11 Ductular cholestasis.

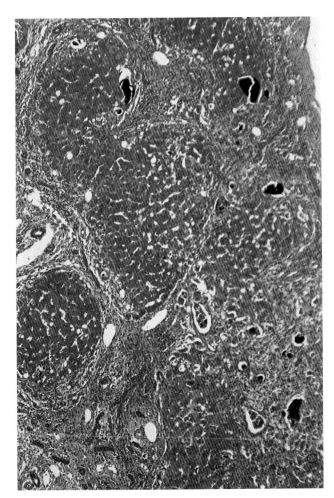

2.10 Intrahepatic cholestasis in cirrhosis.

2.11 Ductular cholestasis

Cholestatic jaundice may be a feature of certain severe illnesses not primarily hepatobiliary in type, e.g. following major abdominal surgery, septicemia and shock. The cause is probably multifactorial including hemolysis with production of excessive bilirubin for conjugation in the liver, failure of hepatocytes to excrete this product, and condensation of bile through loss of fluid. Histological examination may show centrilobular cholestasis (**2.2**, **2.3**), or there may be plugs of bile in ductules, as in this case of cardiogenic shock. Ischemic centrilobular necrosis is evident also in this case (below). ×113 Hematoxylin and eosin.

2.12 Large bile duct obstruction and dilatation

This patient had obstructive jaundice due to cholangio-carcinoma arising at the porta hepatis and spreading within the liver as multiple pale nodules seen in the lower part of the picture. Above, there are several bile-stained cavities which represent grossly dilated intrahepatic bile ducts.

2.13 Widening of portal tract in extrahepatic bile duct obstruction

There is inflammatory edema and vascular dilatation of this portal tract and a tendency to a concentric arrangement of connective tissue cells around its bile duct which has a damaged epithelial lining. Inflammatory cells are fairly numerous in the portal area and adjacent parenchyma. There are foci of cholestasis with dark plugs of bile pigment in bile capillaries (arrows). × 59 Hematoxylin and eosin.

2.14 Dilatation of interlobular duct from extrahepatic bile duct obstruction

There is obvious dilatation of the interlobular duct with thinning or loss of its epithelial lining and inspissated bile in the lumen. It is surrounded by concentric bands of fibrous tissue. Bile ductular proliferation is also evident (arrow). × 56 Hematoxylin and eosin.

2.15 Obstruction of large bile duct with epithelial proliferation

Mitotic activity is prominent in the epithelial lining of this intrahepatic septal duct. From a case of common bile duct obstruction by calculus. × 187 Hematoxylin and eosin.

2.16 Obstruction of large bile duct with epithelial proliferation

This autopsy specimen shows inflammatory edema of a septum. It contains a large septal duct with papilliform proliferation of its epithelial lining partly desquamated into the lumen, where there is also some inspissated bile. Bile ductular proliferation is evident at the inner margin of the septum. × 45 Hematoxylin and eosin.

2.17 Proliferation of bile ductules associated with large duct obstruction

The inflamed portal tract has numerous bile ductular structures at its junction with adjacent liver parenchyma. These may arise both by proliferation of pre-existing ductules and by metaplasia of adjacent hepatocytes as some appear to be continuous with

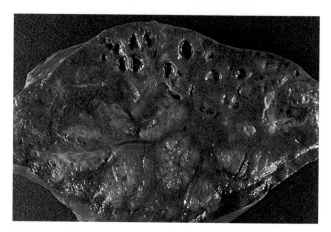

2.12 Large bile duct obstruction and dilatation.

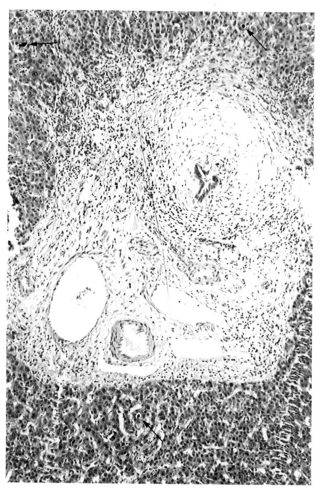

2.13 Widening of portal tract in extrahepatic bile duct obstruction.

liver cell plates. Intrahepatic cholestasis is prominent. Ductular proliferation is a common feature of large duct obstruction, and can be produced experimentally by ligation of the common bile duct. Lesser degrees may be seen in other forms of chronic liver disease. × 134 Hematoxylin and eosin.

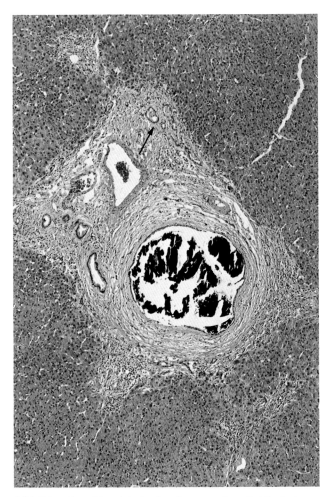

2.14 Dilatation of interlobular duct from extrahepatic bile duct obstruction.

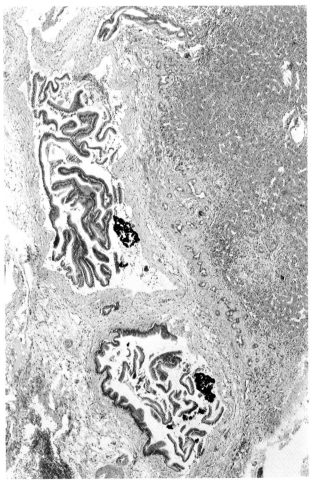

2.16 Obstruction of large bile duct with epithelial proliferation.

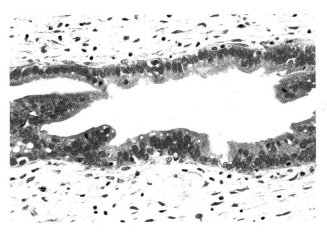

2.15 Obstruction of large bile duct with epithelial proliferation.

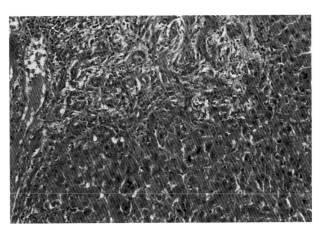

2.17 Proliferation of bile ductules associated with large duct obstruction.

2.18 Acute cholangitis from obstruction of a large bile duct

Acute inflammatory cells are seen in the lumens and walls of small bile ducts which are not dilated. While this can occur in other conditions such as drug-induced cholestatic hepatitis and primary biliary cirrhosis, the widening of the portal tract with inflammatory edema is suggestive of the large duct obstruction which was present in this case. × 167 Hematoxylin and eosin.

2.19 Suppurative cholangiohepatitis from obstruction of a large bile duct

Suppuration has developed in the portal tract (below) and spread into the adjacent liver parenchyma. The surviving bile duct contains acute inflammatory cells. Macrophages are numerous at the periphery of the lesion where fibroblastic activity can also be seen. There is centrilobular cholestasis (above). × 71 Hematoxylin and eosin.

2.20 Subacute cholangiohepatitis with xanthoma cells

There is inflammation in and around a small duct showing epithelial cell proliferation. Many macrophages have ingested lipid which gives their cytoplasm a foamy appearance (xanthoma cells). Occasionally in cases of biliary disease associated with large duct obstruction there are discrete collections of macrophages with or without multinucleated giant cells situated within the liver parenchyma. Accordingly, biliary obstruction should be considered in the differential diagnosis of granulomatous hepatitis (**8.6**). × 187 Hematoxylin and eosin.

2.21 Subacute cholangiohepatitis with feathery degeneration of hepatocytes

Feathery degeneration is seen in biliary disease and affects groups of hepatocytes adjacent to inflamed portal tracts. The cytoplasm of the damaged cells stains faintly and contains fine wisps of material which has been likened to feathers. The affected cells are often bile-stained although this is not prominent in this picture. There is often a close resemblance to, and association with, xanthoma cells and it may not always be possible to distinguish between the two cell types. × 234 Hematoxylin and eosin.

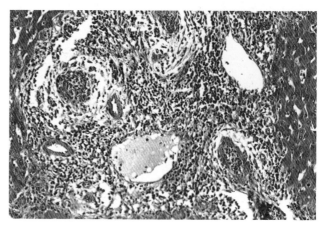

2.18 Acute cholangitis from obstruction of a large bile duct.

2.22 Bile infarct

There is a focus of fibrinoid necrosis surrounded by atrophic hepatocytes and adjacent to a small portal tract (right) which is infiltrated by lymphocytes. Necrosis in these lesions involves mesenchymal cells as well as hepatocytes. Xanthoma cells are seen at the margin of the lesion. Bile infarcts are usually bile-stained but this is not evident here. They may be present in a variety of biliary diseases and when prominent they are usually associated with a large bile duct obstruction. × 117 Hematoxylin and eosin.

2.23 Bile lake

A bile lake is formed by seepage of bile pigment into a bile infarct. In this example there is prominent inspissated pigment surrounded by a cuff of macrophages. Note again the position of the lesion in close proximity to a portal tract on the right, where there is some bile-ductular proliferation. × 75 Hematoxylin and eosin.

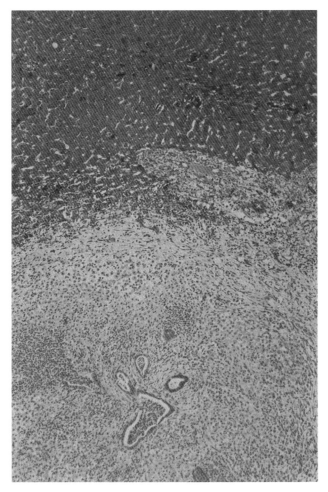

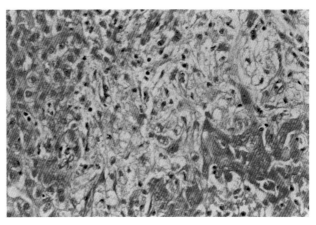

2.21 Subacute cholangiohepatitis with feathery degeneration of hepatocytes.

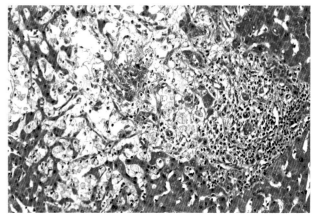

2.22 Bile infarct.

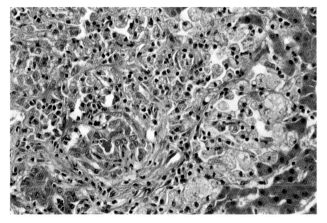

2.19 Suppurative cholangiohepatitis from obstruction of a large bile duct.

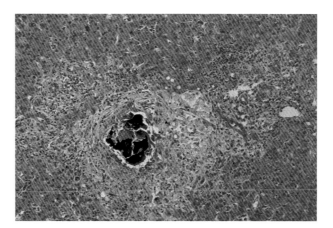

2.20 Subacute cholangiohepatitis with xanthoma cells.

2.23 Bile lake.

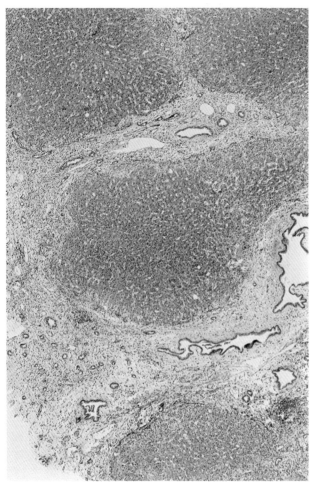

2.24 Chronic cholangiohepatitis with bridging portal fibrosis.

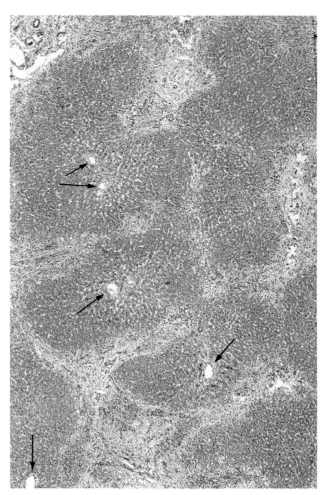

2.25 Developing secondary biliary cirrhosis.

2.24 Chronic cholangiohepatitis with bridging portal fibrosis

Bands of fibrous tissue extend between adjacent portal tracts where there is chronic inflammation and bile-ductular proliferation. A large septal duct is dilated. This is from a case of biliary obstruction due to carcinoma of head of pancreas. × 36 Hematoxylin and eosin.

2.25 Developing secondary biliary cirrhosis

In this case failure to relieve common bile duct obstruction caused by a fibrous stricture has resulted in chronic persistent cholangiohepatitis with production of somewhat edematous fibrous tissue. As it spreads the fibrous tissue delineates the periphery of liver lobules (monolobular fibrosis or cirrhosis) and it is evident that the centres of these lobules, each with a centrilobular venule (arrows), are unaffected by fibrosis. True cirrhosis with more obvious nodular proliferation of surviving parenchyma may supervene. × 36 Hematoxylin and eosin.

2.26 Sclerosing cholangitis with dilatation of intrahepatic bile ducts

This patient had idiopathic sclerosing cholangitis which extended distally from the middle of his common bile duct into both main liver lobes especially the left. This section taken from the left lobe at autopsy shows very gross dilatation of septal bile ducts which contain inspissated bile. Other sections showed fibrous obliteration of smaller ducts. × 30 Hematoxylin and eosin.

2.27 Sclerosing cholangitis with fibrous obliteration of intrahepatic bile ducts

Another field from the case illustrated in **2.26**. This shows a portal tract with an interlobular bile duct completely obliterated by fibrous tissue (arrow). Sclerosing cholangitis more commonly complicates chronic inflammatory bowel disease, especially ulcerative colitis. × 106 Hematoxylin and eosin.

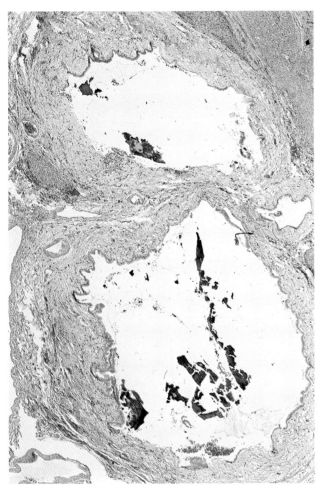

2.26 Sclerosing cholangitis with dilatation of intrahepatic bile ducts.

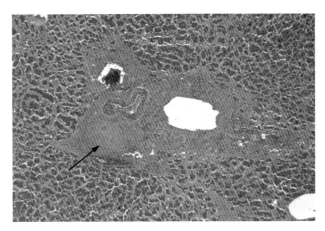

2.27 Sclerosing cholangitis with fibrous obliteration of intrahepatic bile ducts.

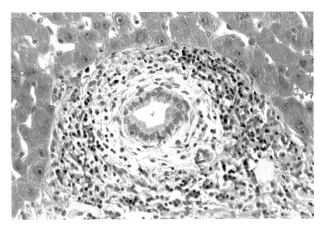

2.28 Pericholangitis complicating chronic inflammatory bowel disease.

2.28 Pericholangitis complicating chronic inflammatory bowel disease

This liver biopsy from a case of ulcerative colitis shows a small interlobular bile duct surrounded by a cuff of inflammatory edema with a lymphocytic infiltrate. Granulomas may be found adjacent to these inflamed ducts when the resemblance to primary biliary cirrhosis can be very close. In the latter condition the affected bile ducts are often somewhat larger and the lymphocyte infiltration more dense (**7.15**). × 140 Hematoxylin and eosin.

2.29 Liver in Crohn's disease

There is a rather poorly formed granuloma related to a small bile duct lined by degenerate epithelium. Lymphocytes and plasma cells are seen but the infiltrate is not dense. Crohn's disease is a recognized cause of granulomatous hepatitis but the lesion is found in only a minority of cases. Moreover, granulomas may be found occasionally in other forms of chronic colitis. × 187 Hematoxylin and eosin.

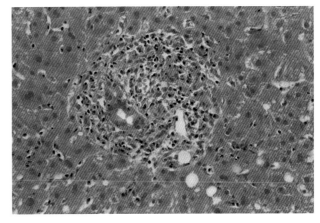

2.29 Liver in Crohn's disease.

CHAPTER 3

Vascular Disorders

3.1 Polyarteritis involving branches of the hepatic artery

There is fibrinoid necrosis of the wall of the artery (small arrow) which is surrounded by a broad zone of acute inflammatory edema. This is continuous below with an area of hepatic necrosis in which can be detected the outlines of other vessels, one containing organizing thrombus (large arrow). Branches of the hepatic artery are not infrequently involved in polyarteritis nodosa. Occasionally there is an association with hepatitis B infection and drug sensitivity. The lesions are often multiple and may cause gross infarction of liver. × 71 Hematoxylin and eosin.

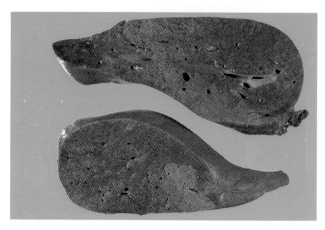

3.2 Infarction of liver.

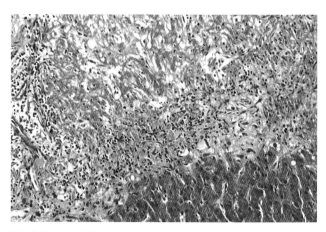

3.3 Infarction of liver.

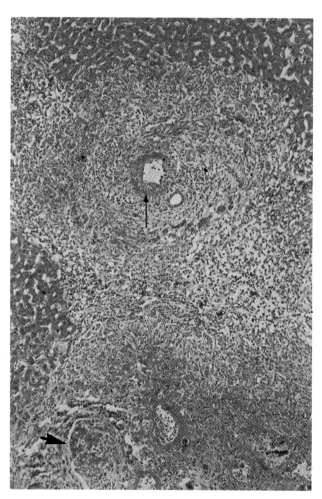

3.1 Polyarteritis involving branches of the hepatic artery.

3.2 Infarction of liver

These are two slices of liver from a case of accidental surgical ligation of the hepatic artery distal to the origin of the right gastric artery. There are large irregular pale areas of massive necrosis. The remainder of the liver appears acutely congested and had microscopic features of centrilobular zonal necrosis.

3.3 Infarction of liver

There is coagulative necrosis of parenchyma separated from viable hepatic tissue by a thin band of organization. The infarct was a consequence of abdominal trauma sustained about three days before the biopsy was obtained. × 117 Hematoxylin and eosin.

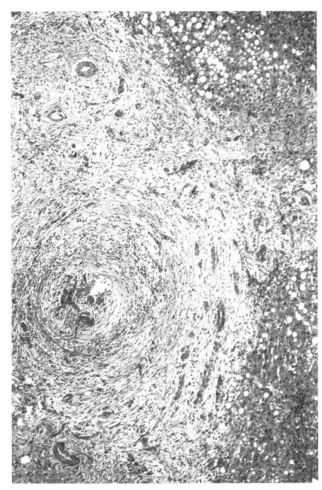

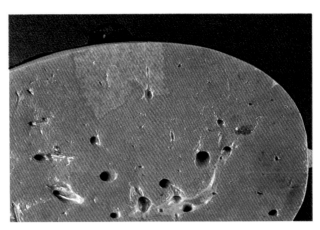

3.5 Zahn's infarct of liver.

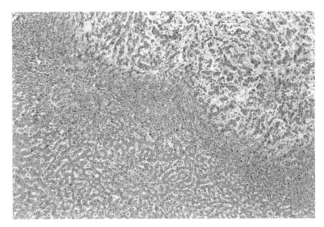

3.4 Intrahepatic portal venous thrombosis.

3.6 Zahn's infarct.

3.4 Intrahepatic portal venous thrombosis

The lumen of a medium-sized portal vein is almost occluded by thrombus undergoing organization. There is a wide margin of inflammatory edema and a concentric arrangement of fibroblasts round the occluded vessel. Proliferation of bile ductules is evident. From a case of common bile duct stricture complicated by suppurative cholangitis and extensive portal venous thrombosis. × 71 Hematoxylin and eosin.

3.5 Zahn's infarct of liver

A pale, well-defined rectangular area under the capsule consists of hepatocytes affected by fatty change. The lesion was associated with thrombosis of adjacent small portal veins. More commonly these lesions, which result from portal or hepatic venous obstruction, are dull red in colour and triangular in shape with their base at the liver capsule.

3.6 Zahn's infarct

This shows part of a typical example (above right) consisting of atrophic hepatocytes separated by dilated sinusoids. × 75 Hematoxylin and eosin.

3.7 Acute venous congestion

The liver in acute circulatory failure, in this case caused by myocardial infarction. There is intense congestion which exaggerates the normal lobular pattern. A similar change may be found in patients dying in a state of shock, especially when this had persisted for more than one day.

3.8 Acute congestion superimposed on chronic circulatory failure

There is dilatation of sinusoids with severe congestion of these channels adjacent to two centrilobular veins where the adjacent hepatocytes have undergone atrophy or necrosis. The intervening indistinct nodularity of the parenchyma without fibrosis is more typical of an underlying chronic circulatory insufficiency and is more clearly illustrated in **3.13**. ×71 Hematoxylin and eosin.

3.9 Empty dilated sinusoids in circulatory failure

Despite severe hepatic congestion many sinusoids are empty although dilated, erythrocytes being present within Disse's space which exists between sinusoidal lining cells with small flat nuclei, and hepatocytes, many of which are atrophic or have disappeared. This is an infrequent finding in venous congestion of liver. ×187 Hematoxylin and eosin.

3.10 Chronic venous congestion

The cut surface of the liver presents the typical nutmeg appearance of chronic venous congestion. The contrast between the dark congested centrilobular zones and the paler peripheral areas can be more exaggerated than this when the latter undergo fatty change. Fatty change, however, is a variable feature. Nutmeg liver is found particularly in cases of prolonged right-sided cardiac failure, as in mitral stenosis.

3.11 Chronic venous congestion

There is dilatation and congestion of many sinusoids with loss of centrilobular hepatocytes. Note the absence of any inflammatory reaction, although fibrosis may ensue in the congested areas from active fibrogenesis or condensation of pre-existing stroma. This form of centrilobular zonal necrosis is rarely seen in needle aspiration specimens as the diagnostic procedure is not usually undertaken in patients suffering from cardiac failure. In larger autopsy specimens coalescence of adjacent centrilobular necrotic zones may be seen. ×71 Hematoxylin and eosin.

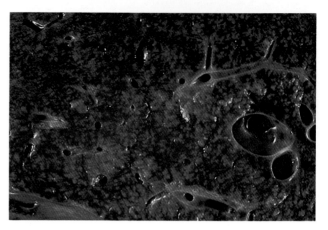

3.7 Acute venous congestion.

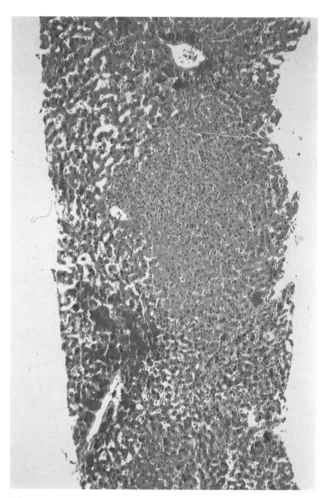

3.8 Acute congestion superimposed on chronic circulatory failure.

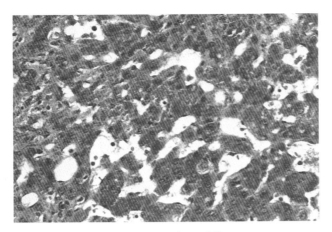

3.9 Empty dilated sinusoids in circulatory failure.

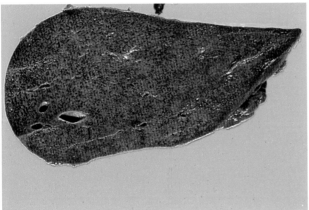

3.10 Chronic venous congestion.

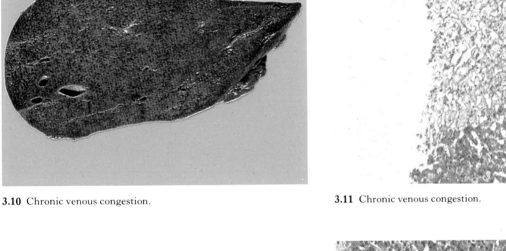

3.11 Chronic venous congestion.

3.12 Cholestasis in circulatory failure

A small plug of dark bile (arrow) and a little intra-cellular bile pigment are seen in association with sinusoidal congestion. Cholestasis may be a feature of acute or chronic circulatory failure and has been particularly noted in cases induced by heat stroke. Jaundice arising in patients with cardiac failure is more frequently non-cholestatic and the result of excess bilirubin production in hemorrhagic pulmonary infarcts. × 117 Hematoxylin and eosin.

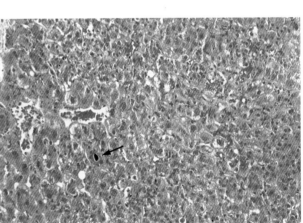

3.12 Cholestasis in circulatory failure.

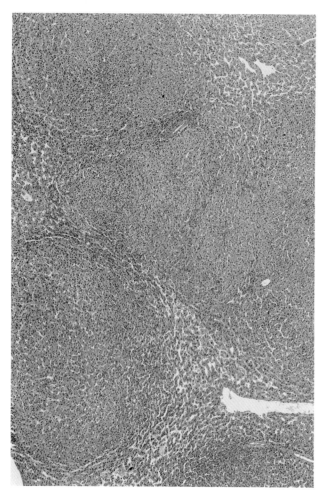

3.13 Nodular regenerative hyperplasia.

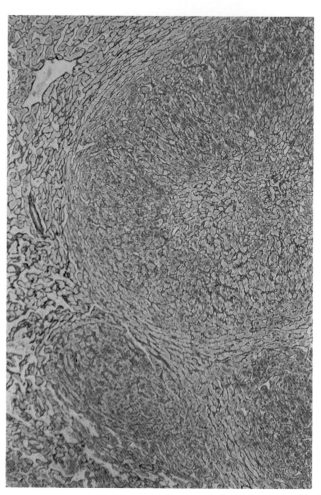

3.14 Nodular regenerative hyperplasia.

3.13 Nodular regenerative hyperplasia

The liver consists of small nodules of parenchyma separated by normal cords of liver cells and dilated sinusoids. There is no fibrosis. This appearance is found usually in patients with chronic circulatory impairment but a similar condition has been described in Felty's syndrome and in association with other manifestations of rheumatoid disease. Anabolic steroid therapy has also been implicated in its development. Nodularity occurs throughout the liver and may cause portal hypertension. The condition is probably different from partial nodular transformation of liver (11.16) which is usually most prominent in the region of the porta hepatis and which may be a developmental anomaly. × 36 Hematoxylin and eosin.

3.14 Nodular regenerative hyperplasia

This reticulin preparation shows clearly the absence of fibrosis, there being no more than minimal condensation of pre-existing stroma at the margins of nodules. Within each nodule the black reticulin fibres which outline sinusoidal walls are very thin. × 71 Reticulin stain.

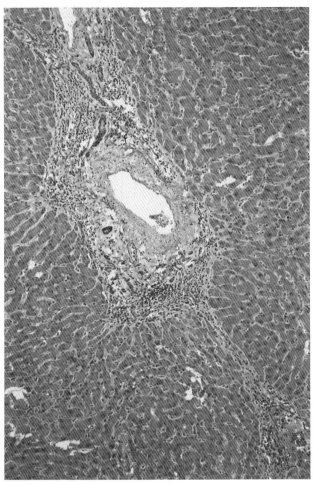

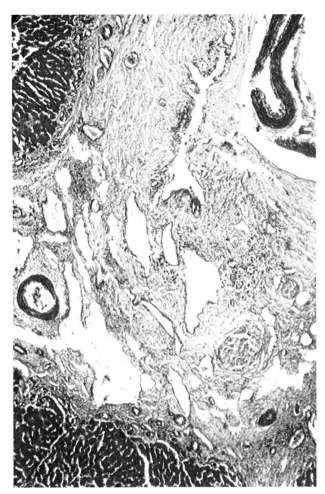

3.15 Non-cirrhotic idiopathic portal fibrosis.

3.16 Cavernomatous transformation of portal vein.

3.15 Non-cirrhotic idiopathic portal fibrosis

There is chronic inflammation of the portal tract with fibrosis extending downwards and to the right as a thin fibrous septum. The medium-sized portal vein has a thick wall and thrombosis can occur in such vessels. These fibrotic and vascular changes are distributed in an irregular fashion within the liver and are associated with portal hypertension. The cause is unknown but some are related to ingestion of arsenic, copper sulphate, vinyl chloride or thorotrast. Some early reports of idiopathic cases originated in India. Because of this and the associated splenomegaly due to portal hypertension, the condition has also been called 'tropical splenomegaly', but this should not be confused with tropical splenomegaly synonymous with 'big spleen disease' which is related to malaria (**8.21**). × 88 Hematoxylin and eosin.

3.16 Cavernomatous transformation of portal vein

This section from the porta hepatis shows a collection of small vessels which replaced the portal vein. This may be a developmental anomaly or a late consequence of venous thrombosis initiated by umbilical vein catheterization which is undertaken in neonates for various therapeutic procedures. It is a cause of portal hypertension, especially in children. × 45 Masson's trichrome stain.

3.17 Budd–Chiari syndrome

The lumen of the inferior vena cava is open and reveals the ostium of a large hepatic vein which is greatly reduced by a web of fibrous tissue. A recent thrombus runs between two small fenestrations in this web (arrow). The liver was acutely congested and had features of cardiac fibrosis.

3.18 Budd–Chiari syndrome

The same lesion illustrated in **3.17** cut to show more clearly the fibrous web (arrow) at the ostium of the hepatic vein. Fibrin lines the wall of this vessel within the liver.

3.19 Budd–Chiari syndrome

Another case showing complete occlusion of an hepatic vein by organized thrombus which includes some congested capillary channels. The lumen of the inferior vena cava is situated above. × 33 Hematoxylin and eosin.

3.20 Veno-occlusive disease

The central hepatic vein shows proliferation of loose subendothelial connective tissue. This process can advance to complete occlusion of the lumen of the vein but there is no thrombosis. These cases suffer from portal hypertension with ascites, and death is often due to hematemesis. Veno-occlusive disease is found in various parts of the world and is endemic in the Caribbean, especially among children in whom it relates to ingestion of herbal medicines and teas containing pyrrolizidine alkaloids. Various other toxins, e.g. urethane (**4.40**) and irradiation, may cause similar hepatic lesions. × 117 Hematoxylin and eosin.

3.21 Veno-occlusive disease

There is involvement of a large interlobular vein by subintimal fibrosis. Part of the adjacent hepatic tissue shows severe congestion and loss of centrilobular liver cells. Involvement of larger veins is atypical, at least in the Caribbean cases. However, this specimen was unusual, coming from an adult living in Scotland who had an addiction to herbal teas which she consumed in large amounts, and from some samples of which pyrrolizidine alkaloids were recovered. × 75 Hematoxylin and eosin.

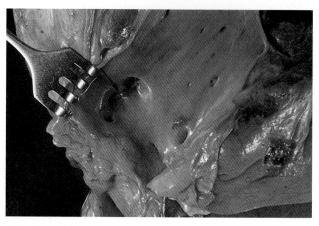

3.17 Budd–Chiari syndrome.

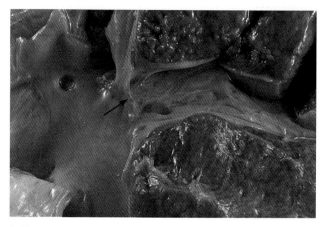

3.18 Budd–Chiari syndrome.

3.22 Hepatic vein thrombosis in leukemia

This is from a case of fatal chronic myeloid leukemia and many leukemic cells are present within sinusoids. A recent thrombus fills the lumen of the hepatic vein and is one of the many similar lesions found throughout the liver. Thrombosis did not extend to larger hepatic veins. Similar lesions may arise in the liver in a variety of blood coagulation disorders. × 87 Hematoxylin and eosin.

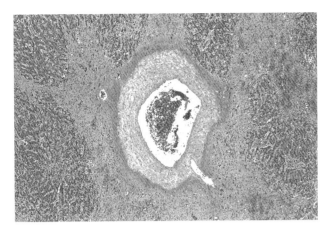

3.21 Veno-occlusive disease.

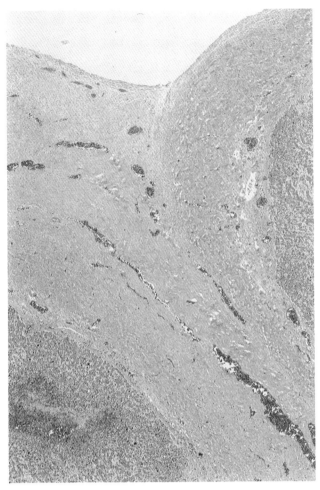

3.19 Budd–Chiari syndrome.

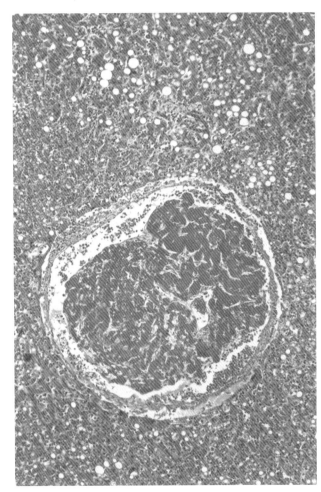

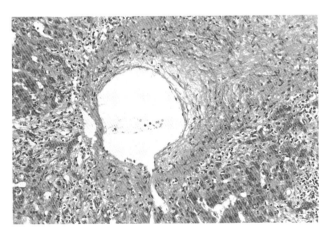

3.20 Veno-occlusive disease.

3.22 Hepatic vein thrombosis in leukemia.

3.23 Cardiac fibrosis ('cirrhosis')

There is some exaggeration of the lobular pattern through hypertrophy of pale surviving parenchyma separated by darker bands of fibrous tissue which radiate from foci of congestion. From a case of long-standing mitral stenosis.

3.24 Cardiac fibrosis with reversed lobulation

Adjacent centrilobular zones are linked by pale fibrous tissue. This results in 'reversed lobulation', with a portal tract in the centre of each pseudolobule, as illustrated here. Hepatocytes disappear from the fibrotic zones or persist as small acinar structures which may be mistaken for proliferating bile ductules (arrows). Sinusoidal dilatation is prominent. It is doubtful whether true cirrhosis with distinct nodular hyperplasia of surviving parenchyma ever occurs in such cases. × 58 Hematoxylin and eosin.

3.25 Cardiac fibrosis

The centrilobular zone on the left contains several dilated capillaries probably derived from sinusoids and much red staining fibrous tissue. There are a few small acinar structures lined by cuboidal epithelium which are the residue of hepatocytes in this zone; in the centre of the field some of these appear to be in continuity with liver cell plates. × 187 Van Gieson's stain and hematoxylin.

3.26 Liver in eclampsia

There is hemorrhagic necrosis. This can be extensive and distributed irregularly in the liver, but smaller lesions are usually periportal in distribution. In this field the necrotic areas are adjacent to two portal tracts (upper and lower right) while the centrilobular zone (lower left) is unaffected. The condition arises as a manifestation of disseminated intravascular coagulation with focal damage to sinusoidal walls. × 71 Hematoxylin and eosin.

3.27 Liver in eclampsia

Fibrin deposition in the necrotic lesions is a feature of eclampsia. In this damaged periportal zone, fibrin is stained red and erythrocytes are yellow. × 58 Mallory's trichrome stain.

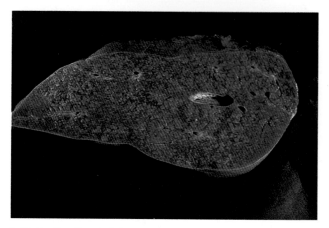

3.23 Cardiac fibrosis ('cirrhosis').

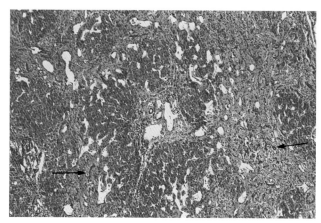

3.24 Cardiac fibrosis with reversed lobulation.

3.28 Liver in shock

Centrilobular congestion and necrosis may be found in shock from a variety of causes. Infiltration of these zones with acute inflammatory cells is an additional feature, especially in biopsies obtained during laparotomy when it may be aggravated by minor surgical trauma. This feature is well illustrated here. Cholestasis in bile capillaries and ductules may also occur (**2.11**). × 113 Hematoxylin and eosin.

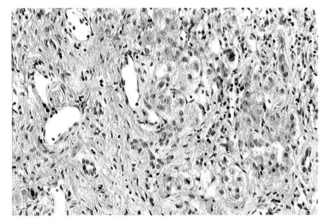

3.25 Cardiac fibrosis.

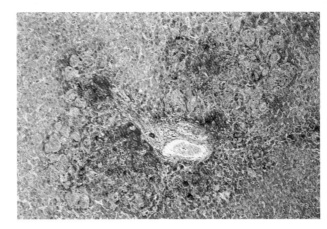

3.27 Liver in eclampsia.

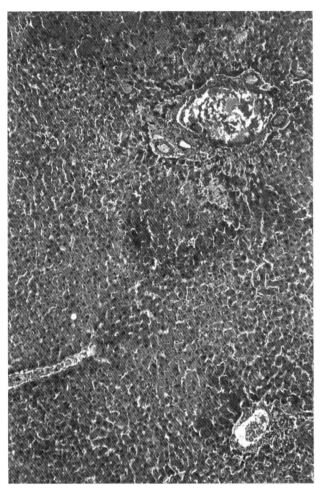

3.26 Liver in eclampsia.

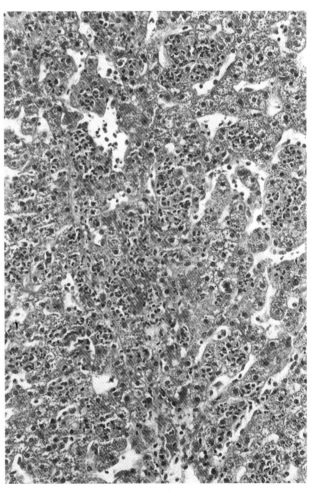

3.28 Liver in shock.

3.29 Ischemia of cirrhotic nodules

A case of post-hepatitis cirrhosis in which some of the nodules of regenerating parenchyma are pale because of ischemic necrosis (centre left). The blood supply to cirrhotic nodules is often precarious and ischemia will be enhanced by episodes of esophageal hemorrhage. Necrosis should not be attributed to persistence of the initial cause of liver damage.

3.30 Ischemia of cirrhotic nodules

When ischemia is less severe it may cause fatty change rather than necrosis. It is most marked in the centres of nodules where oxygen deprivation is greatest, a distribution illustrated in this example of macronodular cirrhosis. It should not be mistaken for alcoholic fatty cirrhosis in which fat is distributed uniformly in the nodular parenchyma (**5.30**). × 45 Hematoxylin and eosin.

3.31 Liver in sickle-cell anemia

There is sinusoidal obstruction caused by clumps of abnormal erythrocytes, fibrin and platelets. Some of this material has been ingested by Kupffer cells. The condition occurs throughout the liver lobules and may give rise to foci of hepatocyte degeneration and necrosis. This liver damage occurs in the homozygotic (SS) form of the disease and may be mistaken clinically for viral hepatitis. × 146 Hematoxylin and eosin.

3.32 Liver in sickle cell anemia

There is phagocytosis of sickle cells by Kupffer cells which are grossly distended as a result of this activity. × 300 Hematoxylin and eosin.

3.33 Peliosis hepatis

Blood-filled cysts measuring up to 1 cm in diameter are scattered in a haphazard fashion throughout the liver. They have no distinct cellular lining and may communicate with sinusoids. Blood in the cysts can undergo thrombosis and organization with formation of small stellate scars (top right). Peliosis hepatis is a rare disease associated with wasting conditions such as tuberculosis and may be aggravated by administration of steroids. This specimen was from a case of advanced ovarian cancer treated with progesterone. Somewhat similar lesions may occur in hairy-cell leukemia. × 35 Hematoxylin and eosin.

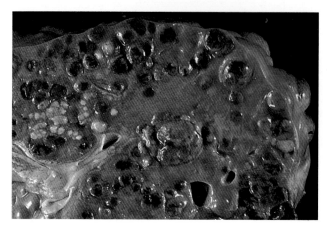

3.29 Ischemia of cirrhotic nodules.

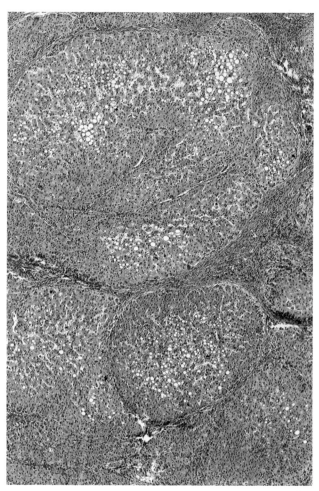

3.30 Ischemia of cirrhotic nodules.

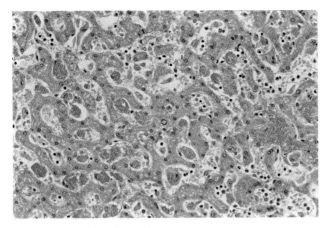

3.31 Liver in sickle-cell anemia.

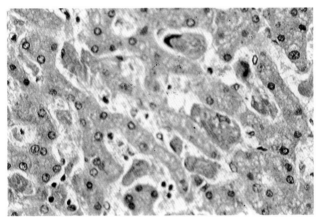

3.32 Liver in sickle cell anemia.

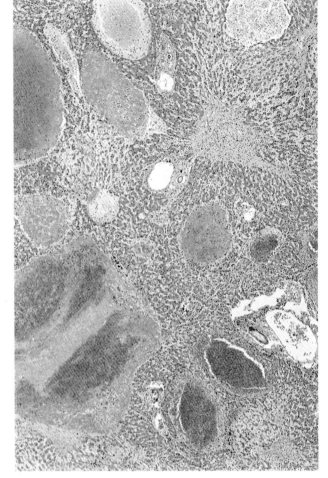

3.33 Peliosis hepatis.

3.34 Peliosis hepatis

Parts of two cysts are seen each containing erythrocytes, which are stained yellow, and fibrin, which is stained red. Note that the cyst walls have no distinct endothelial lining and no blue staining connective tissue capsule. ×117 Martius scarlet blue.

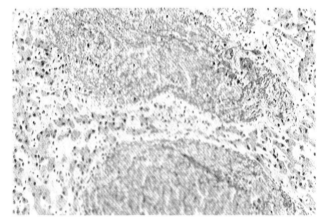

3.34 Peliosis hepatis.

3.35 Hereditary hemorrhagic telangiectasia (Rendu–Osler–Weber syndrome)

The liver can be a site for the multiple telangiectatic lesions which occur in the syndrome, although it is unusual for them to produce clinical evidence of hepatic disease, being manifest more frequently at other sites, such as skin or alimentary tract. In the liver the lesions may be in the form of discrete hemangiomas of variable size, sometimes associated with prominent blood vessels in portal tracts. The enlarged portal tract in the centre of this field contains blood vessels which appear related to the two adjacent cavernous hemangiomas at its upper and lower margins. × 30 Hematoxylin and eosin.

3.36 Hereditary hemorrhagic telangiectasia

Telangiectasia without limiting fibrosis is another feature of the disease. Two such lesions are present in this field. A large cavernous hemangioma, about 10 cm in diameter, was present elsewhere in the liver. × 30 Hematoxylin and eosin.

3.37 Hereditary hemorrhagic telangiectasia

The vascular lesions may become extensive and fibrotic, producing a type of cirrhosis. In this example the liver parenchyma is traversed by bands of fibrous tissue in which are numerous blood vascular channels. These may include arterio-venous fistulas demonstrable by angiography and the cause of a continuous bruit and palpable thrill in an enlarged liver. While this cirrhosis is a distinct entity there is also an association between the syndrome and certain cases of primary biliary cirrhosis and chronic active hepatitis. The development of hepatocellular carcinoma is also recorded. × 30 Martius-scarlet-blue.

3.38 Hereditary hemorrhagic telangiectasia

A higher magnification of part of the lesion shown in **3.37**. There are two small arterioles with thick muscular walls (right) and a third (centre left). Several dilated venous channels and capillaries are present also. These vessels are surrounded by blue fibrous tissue which has entrapped small groups of hepatocytes. × 117 Martius-scarlet-blue.

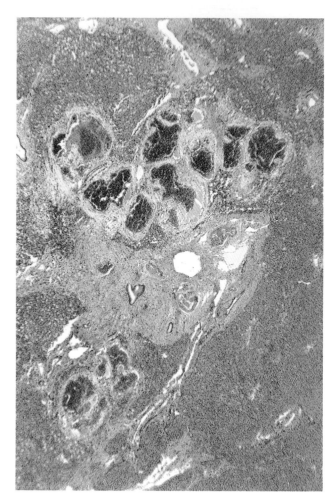

3.35 Hereditary hemorrhagic telangiectasia (Rendu–Osler–Weber syndrome).

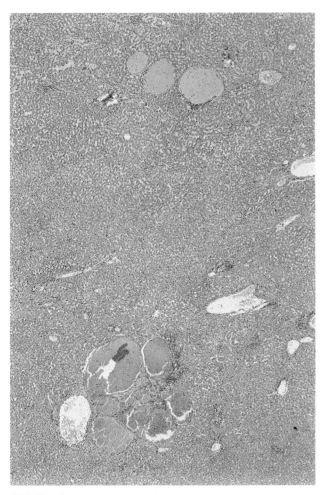

3.36 Hereditary hemorrhagic telangiectasia.

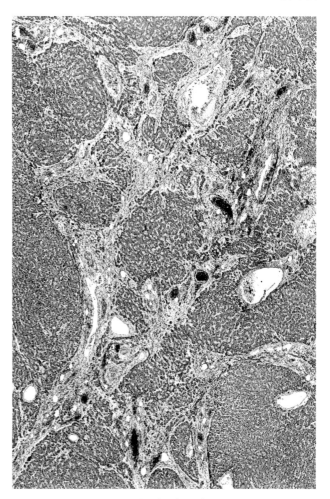

3.37 Hereditary hemorrhagic telangiectasia.

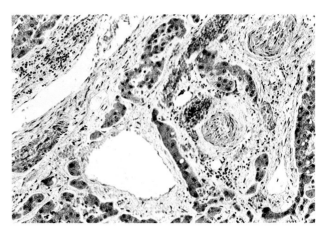

3.38 Hereditary hemorrhagic telangiectasia.

CHAPTER 4

Toxins, Drugs and Physical Agents

4.1 to **4.14** inclusive are examples of experimentally-induced liver injury in small rodents. They are intended to supplement the illustrations of certain predictable injuries, the development of which cannot be followed so readily in human material.

4.1 Acute carbon tetrachloride-induced injury

The liver of a young adult male mouse one day after the administration of a sublethal dose of carbon tetrachloride. The presence of zonal necrosis exaggerates the lobular pattern of the organ, each damaged centrilobular area being darker than the surviving peripheral parenchyma where fatty change is largely responsible for the pallor.

4.2 Acute carbon tetrachloride-induced injury

A section of mouse liver treated by Giemsa's stain to reveal dark coarse basophil granules in the cytoplasm of undamaged hepatocytes (lower centre). Basophil granules are seen less clearly in sections stained with hematoxylin and eosin. They represent profiles of rough endoplasmic reticulum and disappear when there is damage to these organelles with dislocation of their ribosomes from membranes, a process which results in impaired protein synthesis. Loss of basophil granules in all centrilobular hepatocytes is evident in this photograph (arrows indicate centrilobular venules). It is an early manifestation of carbon tetrachloride damage, the specimen being obtained within 30 minutes of poisoning. × 117 Giemsa's stain.

4.3 Acute carbon tetrachloride-induced injury

In this mouse liver there is hydropic swelling with loss of purple-stained glycogen in damaged hepatocytes. The distribution of the lesion in the lobules is mid-zonal. Small groups of affected cells are necrotic (arrow). The hepatocyte damage developed within 12 hours of poisoning. It would be followed by necrosis of the centrilobular cells while the periportal hepatocytes would remain viable. × 50 Periodic acid-Schiff method and hematoxylin.

4.4 Acute carbon tetrachloride-induced injury

Twenty-four hours after poisoning with carbon tetrachloride there is a clear pattern of centrilobular necrosis in mouse liver with complete absence of glycogen-containing hepatocytes from the damaged zones. Viable periportal cells retain glycogen but show some cytoplasmic vacuolation due to fatty change. In the necrotic zones the nuclei of undamaged stromal cells are seen and there is a little increase in mesenchymal cells around some centrilobular veins. × 75 Periodic acid-Schiff method, hematoxylin and orange G.

4.5 Acute carbon tetrachloride-induced injury

An autoradiographic preparation of liver of a mouse given radioactive (tritiated) thymidine one hour before killing and two days after carbon tetrachloride. The black granules represent the radioactive marker incorporated into DNA, and are evidence of very recent DNA synthesis among surviving hepatocytes (left) and among mesenchymal cells including vascular endothelium in the necrotic zone (right). Some hepatocytes with labelled nuclei are in mitosis (arrows). × 234 Autoradiograph.

4.6 Acute carbon tetrachloride-induced injury

Five days after poisoning, regeneration of this mouse liver is well advanced, new hepatocytes being derived from the periportal cells which escaped injury. The necrotic debris has been removed by macrophages but numbers of these persist in the centrilobular zones. × 81 Periodic acid-Schiff method, hematoxylin and orange G.

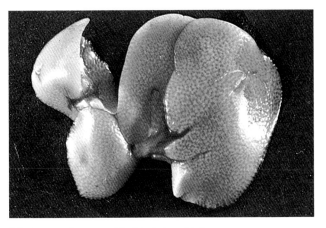

4.1 Acute carbon tetrachloride-induced injury.

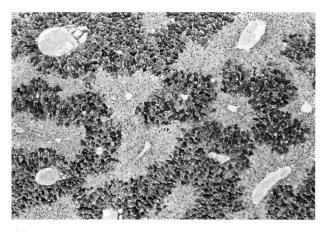

4.4 Acute carbon tetrachloride-induced injury.

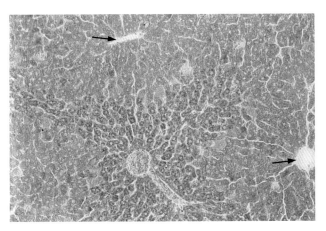

4.2 Acute carbon tetrachloride-induced injury.

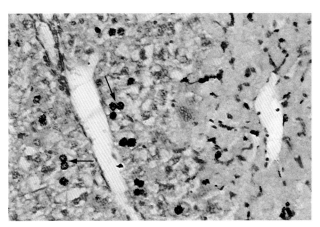

4.5 Acute carbon tetrachloride-induced injury.

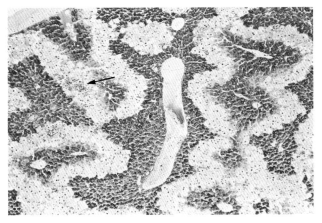

4.3 Acute carbon tetrachloride-induced injury.

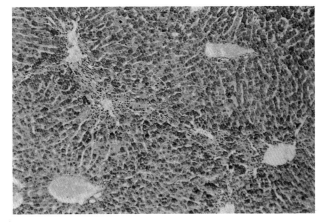

4.6 Acute carbon tetrachloride-induced injury.

4.7 Acute allyl formate-induced injury

There is zonal necrosis of guinea-pig liver which has a periportal distribution, the damaged cells with eosinophilic cytoplasm forming a wide cuff round the portal tract. To the left of this is a centrilobular zone with intact parenchyma. Such a pattern of liver damage is uncommon and may be explained in this instance by the production of toxic metabolites from allyl formate through the action of alcohol dehydrogenase which has a maximal concentration in periportal cells. The majority of predictable liver poisons act like carbon tetrachloride in producing a centrilobular pattern of necrosis. × 47 Hematoxylin and eosin.

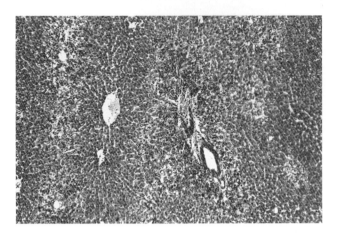

4.7 Acute allyl formate-induced injury.

4.8 Acute bromobenzine-induced injury

Bromobenzine has a rather variable effect on rat liver which depends to some extent on the nutritional state of the animal. In this case it has caused submassive hepatic necrosis involving several adjacent lobules in their entirety; part of such a lesion is shown on the right. In the remainder there is minor damage to mid-zonal cells with loss of glycogen. In some rats given bromobenzine there may be mid-zonal or centrilobular necrosis rather than submassive lesions. × 117 Periodic acid-Schiff method and hematoxylin.

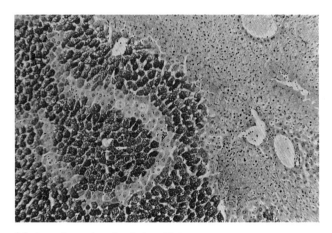

4.8 Acute bromobenzine-induced injury.

4.9 Acute bromobenzine-induced injury

The liver from a rat, 48 hours after poisoning. Extensive areas of pale massive necrosis are seen on the undersurface of the specimen. Necrosis extended into the substance of the organ to a depth of several adjacent lobules.

4.10 Cirrhosis induced by carbon tetrachloride

The liver of a mouse which had received a sublethal dose of carbon tetrachloride by esophageal tube twice weekly for six months. It is clearly cirrhotic.

4.11–4.14 Cirrhosis induced by carbon tetrachloride

Reticulin staining of livers of mice taken at six (**4.11**), twelve (**4.12**), eighteen (**4.13**) and twenty-four (**4.14**) weeks after repeated administration of carbon tetrachloride shows fibrosis of increasing severity. At the early stage there is formation of thin fibrous septa which tend to form bridges between damaged centrilobular zones. Later these septa become thicker and divide the surviving parenchyma into small islands each about the size of a lobule or part of a lobule. **4.14** also illustrates nodular regeneration which is indicative of true cirrhosis. × 47 Reticulin stain.

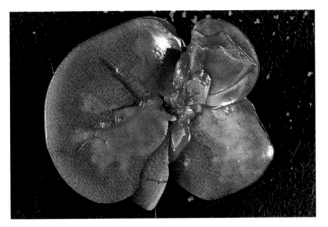

4.9 Acute bromobenzine-induced injury.

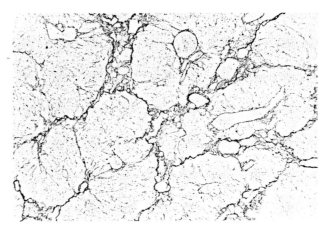

4.12 Cirrhosis induced by carbon tetrachloride.

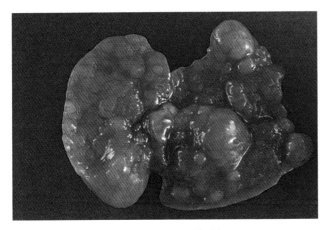

4.10 Cirrhosis induced by carbon tetrachloride.

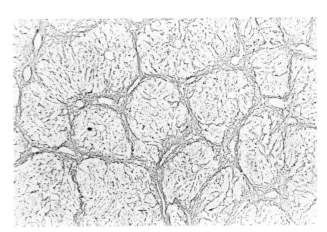

4.13 Cirrhosis induced by carbon tetrachloride.

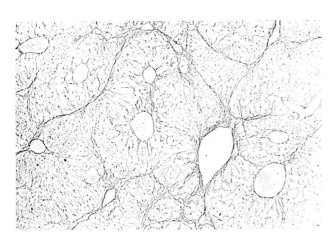

4.11 Cirrhosis induced by carbon tetrachloride.

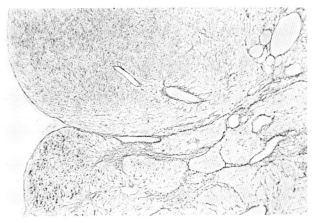

4.14 Cirrhosis induced by carbon tetrachloride.

4.15 Agranular endoplasmic reticulum (AER) hypertrophy

Hepatocytes are slightly enlarged and have dense eosinophilic cytoplasm. Basophil granules representing rough endoplasmic reticulum tend to be displaced to the cell apex adjacent to the bile canaliculus (arrow). There is some resemblance to the ground-glass cells of hepatitis B infection, but AER hypertrophy affects hepatocytes more diffusely and does not have the same fine granular appearance. A number of drugs such as phenobarbitone, steroid hormones and alcohol have this effect on the liver. AER hypertrophy may be accompanied by increased activity of its associated enzymes and this can be beneficial in detoxifying ingested agents. On the other hand the opposite result may ensue if toxicity is due to the metabolic product of a basically harmless substance such as carbon tetrachloride. × 300 Hematoxylin and eosin.

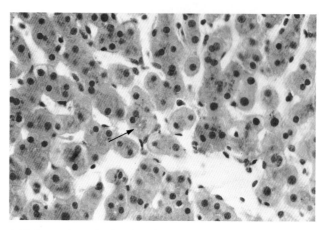

4.15 Agranular endoplasmic reticulum (AER) hypertrophy.

4.16 Acute carbon tetrachloride-induced injury

This shows the liver from a fatal human case of carbon tetrachloride poisoning. There is undue prominence of the lobular pattern, the pale areas being the necrotic centrilobular zones. Fatal carbon tetrachloride injury is unusual in man and occurs most often in association with alcoholism. Zonal necrosis from other causes has a similar appearance.

4.17 Acute carbon tetrachloride-induced injury

Another fatal human case showing well-defined zonal necrosis of the liver, the dark periportal surviving cells representing a minority of each lobule. The lesion is essentially similar to the acute injury in rodents illustrated above. In this case severe renal tubular damage was also contributing to death. Note the absence of any inflammatory response in the liver. × 71 Hematoxylin and eosin.

4.18 Submassive necrosis

Pale necrotic liver occupies much of this field. This was a suicide due to ingestion of a massive dose of tetrachlorethane. In smaller amounts this poison may cause a centrilobular zonal necrosis but with larger doses necrosis extends throughout entire lobules especially at the periphery of the liver.

4.19 Paracetamol-induced liver injury

There is loss of hepatocytes in the centrilobular zone which has dilated central veins. There is macrophage activity in relation to this damage, some of these cells being swollen with ingested brick-red ceroid pigment. Paracetamol is now an important member of that main group of drugs and toxins which can damage the liver in a predictable manner, generally by producing centrilobular zonal necrosis. It is rather less toxic than other poisons in this category such as carbon tetrachloride, chloroform and tannic acid, and liver damage occurs only with gross overdosage. × 75 Hematoxylin and eosin.

4.20 Paracetamol-induced liver injury

Ceroid is a pigmented lipoprotein found within macrophages. It occurs in the livers of man and of experimental animals damaged in a variety of ways, and is often prominent during recovery from drug-induced injury as in this case of paracetamol poisoning. In paraffin sections it stains readily with Sudan stains. × 146 Sudan black and safranin.

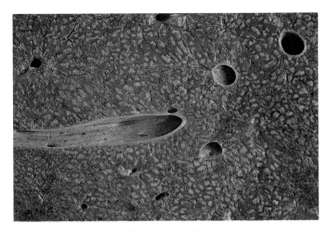

4.16 Acute carbon tetrachloride-induced injury.

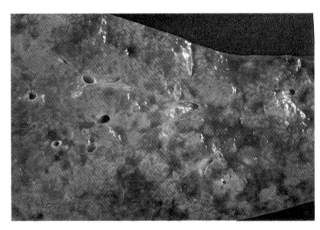

4.18 Submassive necrosis.

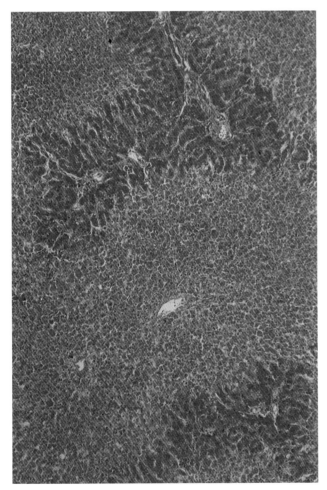

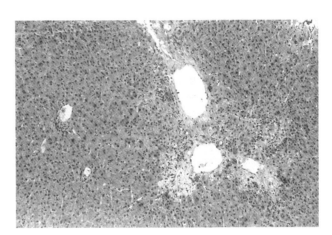

4.19 Paracetamol-induced liver injury.

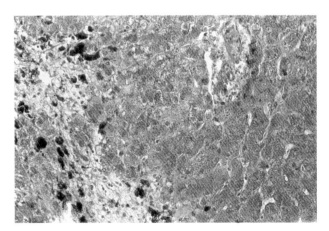

4.17 Acute carbon tetrachloride-induced injury.

4.20 Paracetamol-induced liver injury.

4.21 Phosphorus-induced liver injury

Death occurred from liver failure within a few days of ingestion of yellow phosphorus incorporated in rat poison. The whole liver is pale because of severe fatty change while there is also histological evidence of hepatocyte necrosis with a periportal distribution. In some cases necrosis is inconspicuous, and in these fatty change is most severe in periportal cells.

4.22 Phosphorus-induced liver injury

Another example of acute phosphorus poisoning in a patient dying under similar circumstances. Apart from pallor due to fat there is prominence of the lobular pattern associated with periportal zonal necrosis.

4.23 Periportal zonal necrosis

About half the hepatocytes in this field show acidophilic necrosis and nuclear pyknosis. These are arranged around the portal triad (right). The viable hepatocytes round the central vein (left) are vacuolated because of fine droplet fatty change. This is from a child who also had severe renal damage and who died soon after the administration of a time-expired pentavalent antimony compound wrongly administered in the treatment of schistosomiasis. Severe damage to tissues other than liver is a feature of many of these toxins which act in a predictable fashion on all persons to whom they are given. × 117 Hematoxylin and eosin.

4.24 Tetracycline-induced liver injury

There is fine-droplet fatty change affecting centrilobular and mid-zonal hepatocytes (portal tract on right and centrilobular vein on left of centre). Despite the absence of established hepatic necrosis these patients suffer from severe and sometimes fatal liver injury as in this case. Tetracycline causes liver damage if given in large doses, especially parenterally, or if given to pregnant women and patients with renal insufficiency in whom excretion is impaired. Cholestasis is not a feature of these cases. × 75 Hematoxylin and eosin.

4.25 Acute fatty liver of pregnancy

The same fine-droplet fatty change is seen as in tetracycline liver injury. In this fatal case it extends throughout the entire lobule but is most marked in centrilobular hepatocytes. Congestion of the sinusoids is notable but incidental. While some of the obstetric cases may be associated with tetracycline therapy, the cause in the majority is unknown although probably due to unidentified toxic substances. In contrast to large droplet fatty change which is common and an unimportant cause of liver dysfunction, the microvesicular form as seen here and in other conditions (**4.24, 9.43**) must be regarded as a serious manifestation of liver damage. × 117 Hematoxylin and eosin.

4.26 Post-necrotic scarring of liver

A very coarse form of cirrhosis with extensive deep scarring and irregular nodular regeneration may follow recovery from any severe form of liver injury with extensive destruction of parenchyma. Most commonly these are cases of submassive necrosis resulting from the intake of a predictably injurious agent. Although the cause in this case was unknown the appearances are typical of post-necrotic scarring.

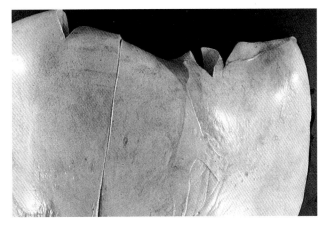

4.21 Phosphorus-induced liver injury.

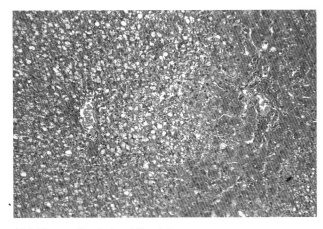

4.24 Tetracycline-induced liver injury.

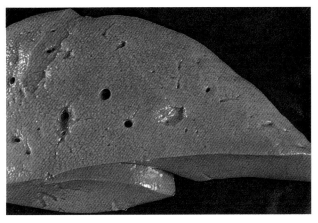

4.22 Phosphorus-induced liver injury.

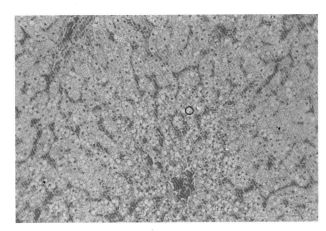

4.25 Acute fatty liver of pregnancy.

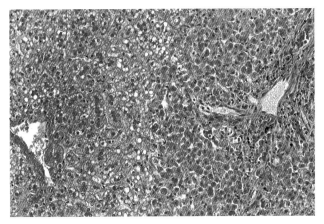

4.23 Periportal zonal necrosis.

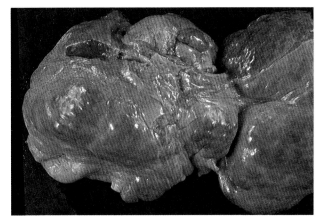

4.26 Post-necrotic scarring of liver.

4.27 Chronic methotrexate-induced liver injury

Hepatocytes show large-droplet fatty change and there is chronic hepatitis with bridging fibrotic lesions between portal tracts and proliferation of bile ductules. The appearances are not unlike chronic alcoholic hepatitis but chronic inflammatory changes tend to be more localized to portal and periportal areas. × 47 Hematoxylin and eosin.

4.28 Chronic methotrexate-induced liver injury

A higher magnification showing piecemeal and focal necrosis of liver cells. Hyaline degeneration as in alcoholic hepatitis of similar severity is not seen. A few hepatocyte nuclei are vacuolated and this is a common feature of methotrexate-induced injury. Chronic hepatitis and even fine cirrhosis can develop in patients taking this drug for long periods, as in the treatment of psoriasis or leukemia. The liver damage should be attributed to continuous administration of the drug rather than the underlying disease for which it is used. The cirrhosis is akin to that induced experimentally by chronic carbon tetrachloride poisoning and is unlike post-necrotic scarring. × 234 Hematoxylin and eosin.

4.29 Drug-induced intrahepatic cholestasis

Centrilobular cholestasis (left) was in this case induced by oral contraceptive steroids. There is no hepatitis and no necrosis. Intrahepatic cholestasis is an uncommon side-effect of taking the contraceptive pill which resolves when it is stopped. There may be a familial susceptibility. Anabolic steroids can have a similar effect in a small minority of patients. × 146 Hematoxylin and eosin.

4.30 Drug-induced cholestatic hepatitis

There is a little cholestasis (top right) and some bile pigment in macrophages. The portal tract (bottom left) is inflamed, being infiltrated by neutrophil polymorphs and a few lymphocytes. These changes were induced by chlorpromazine and resolved on withdrawal of the drug. This is the commonest histological finding in patients who are unusually susceptible to liver damage induced by that main category of drugs possessing non-predictable toxicity. The list of these drugs is long and includes various phenothiazines, thiouracil, para-amino-salicylic acid and oral hypoglycemic agents. × 117 Hematoxylin and eosin.

4.31 Drug-induced cholestatic hepatitis

Another case of chlorpromazine-induced jaundice showing eosinophil leucocytes in the inflamed portal tract. This is a prominent feature in some of these cases and is probably an allergic response to products of tissue damage rather than the drug itself. × 300 Hematoxylin and eosin.

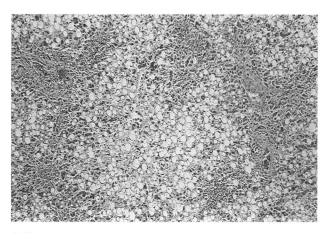

4.27 Chronic methotrexate-induced liver injury.

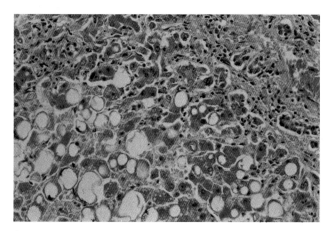

4.28 Chronic methotrexate-induced liver injury.

4.32 Drug-induced chronic biliary disease

This autopsy specimen shows numerous small dark plugs of inspissated bile. Active hepatitis is not prominent but there is extensive fibrosis. The patient gave a three-year history of cholestatic jaundice and had been taking chlorpromazine for the entire period. Such cases may be mistaken on clinical grounds for primary biliary cirrhosis or other forms of biliary disease. × 71 Hematoxylin and eosin.

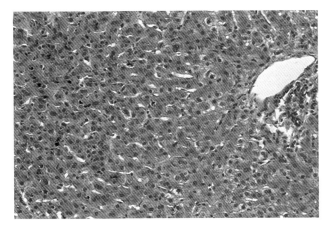

4.29 Drug-induced intrahepatic cholestasis.

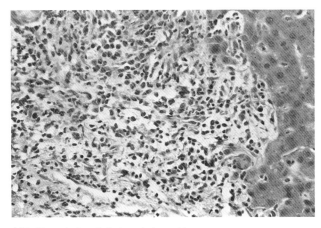

4.31 Drug-induced cholestatic hepatitis.

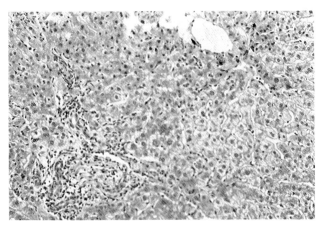

4.30 Drug-induced cholestatic hepatitis.

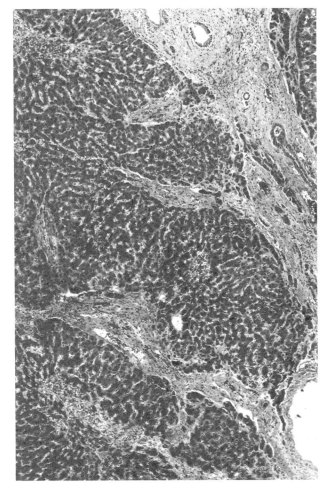

4.32 Drug-induced chronic biliary disease.

4.33 Drug-induced minor hepatitis without cholestasis

There is a mild portal inflammation and a small focus of cell dropout with inflammatory cell accumulation. Such changes, although distributed in an irregular fashion, were sufficient to produce biochemical evidence of liver dysfunction. There is no cholestasis. The overall appearance was that of non-specific reactive hepatitis (**7.8**) and was related in this case to the prolonged ingestion of aspirin for chronic rheumatic disease. A variety of drugs can have this effect which resolves when their use is discontinued. It is important to appreciate that liver damage is due to the drug and not to the basic disease for which it is given. ×113 Hematoxylin and eosin.

4.34 Drug-induced granulomatous hepatitis

There is a lobular hepatitis with small foci of hepatocyte necrosis or dropout and focal collections of inflammatory cells. These include, on the left, two distinct non-caseating granulomas with multinucleated giant cells. It is evident that drug susceptibility must be included among the many causes of granulomatous hepatitis. A number of drugs have been implicated such as allopurinol, phenylbutazone and sulphonamide. Indomethacin was responsible in this case. Other chemicals, such as beryllium, which may be responsible for the production of similar sarcoid-like lesions, can be ingested as a result of industrial exposure. ×63 Hematoxylin and eosin.

4.35 Drug induced granulomatous hepatitis

A higher magnification of the specimen illustrated in **4.34**. There are three discrete non-caseating granulomas. These consist of macrophages including multinucleated giant cells and scanty lymphocytes. ×146 Hematoxylin and eosin.

4.36 Hepatitis from anticonvulsant therapy

There are small foci of hepatocyte necrosis and some surviving liver cells are swollen and hydropic. There is infiltration with chronic inflammatory cells, especially lymphocytes, and Kupffer cells are hyperchromatic. Other parts of this biopsy showed less severe damage with hepatocyte mitotic activity and there were a few indistinct granulomas. The appearances are not unlike those due to infectious mononucleosis and this resemblance is accentuated clinically by generalized lymphadenopathy and circulating atypical lymphocytes. In this case, however, all these changes could be attributed to diphenylhydantoin. ×281 Hematoxylin and eosin.

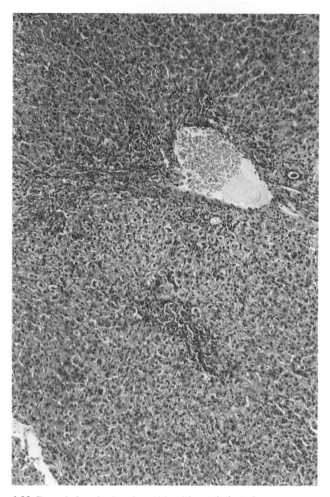

4.33 Drug-induced minor hepatitis without cholestasis.

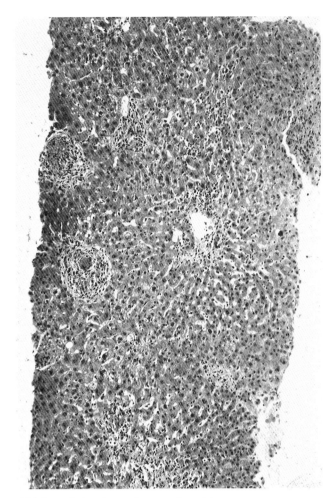

4.34 Drug-induced granulomatous hepatitis.

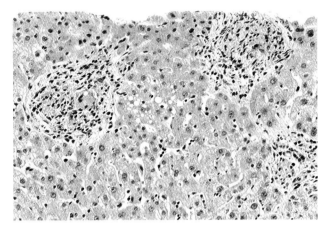

4.35 Drug induced granulomatous hepatitis.

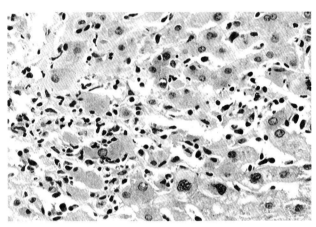

4.36 Hepatitis from anticonvulsant therapy.

4.37 Drug-induced severe hepatitis

A case of halothane hepatitis with portal and lobular inflammation in which the predominant infiltrating cell is the lymphocyte. There is piecemeal loss of hepatocytes and a band of bridging necrosis. Some surviving hepatocytes are swollen and a few show acidophilic necrosis (arrows). The appearances can be mistaken for severe viral hepatitis and a drug etiology should be considered in sporadic cases of this kind. Halothane can cause severe and even fatal liver damage, especially after repeated exposure, and cirrhosis also may develop. For these reasons patients who have experienced halothane liver damage should carry on their person some note of their susceptibility, so that repeated exposure may be avoided. Hepatic necrosis of comparable severity may be induced by another anesthetic, methoxyflurane, and by cinchophen. Less severe but otherwise similar damage can be caused by a number of other drugs including isoniazid and methyldopa. × 117 Hematoxylin and eosin.

4.38 Drug-induced severe hepatitis

Another case of halothane hepatitis showing lobular inflammation and acidophilic necrosis, thereby resembling viral hepatitis. Certain histological features may help to distinguish this drug-induced lesion from virus-induced liver damage such as fatty change, infiltration with eosinophils and better defined centrilobular zonal necrosis, while the severity of hepatitis in the drug cases may be out of keeping with a deceptively mild clinical state. These are inconstant findings and were not present in the cases illustrated. × 117 Hematoxylin and eosin.

4.39 Drug-induced chronic active hepatitis

There is a prominent lymphocytic infiltration of the portal area (bottom left) and hepatic sinusoids. There is destruction of the parenchyma adjacent to the widened portal tract indicative of piecemeal necrosis. Hepatitis in this case was caused by azathioprine. It is accepted that liver damage attributable to certain drugs including some of those mentioned above, such as methyldopa, isoniazid and halothane can progress to chronic active hepatitis with histological features identical with those of the idiopathic cases described in chapter 7. It is important to search for a drug etiology since its withdrawal may be followed by resolution of the hepatitis which might otherwise progress to cirrhosis. × 117 Hematoxylin and eosin.

4.40 Drug-induced veno-occlusive disease

This patient was given urethane as treatment for multiple myeloma. This drug has caused a centrilobular hepatic fibrosis with sclerosis of hepatic venules (upper right) similar to veno-occlusive disease due to pyrrolizidine toxicity (chapter 3). There is severe sinusoidal congestion. Rarely, severe chronic venous congestion of liver can be attributed to hepatic venous thrombosis caused by intake of contraceptive steroids. × 71 Hematoxylin and eosin.

4.41 Disulfiram-induced liver injury

In this example of alcoholic hepatitis some swollen hepatocytes have pale homogeneous cytoplasm (arrows). This change is attributed to disulfiram (antabuse) given as treatment for alcoholism. The cytoplasmic material is PAS-positive and resembles the Lafora bodies which may be present in the liver in myoclonus epilepsy. The affected cells should not be confused with ground-glass cells which are PAS-negative and which give positive staining reactions for hepatitis B infection (**6.23**, **6.24**, **6.25**). × 234 Hematoxylin and eosin.

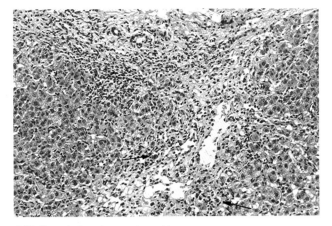

4.37 Drug-induced severe hepatitis.

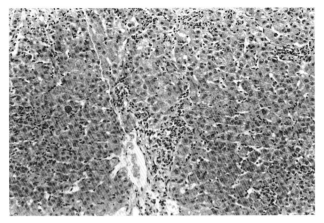

4.38 Drug-induced severe hepatitis.

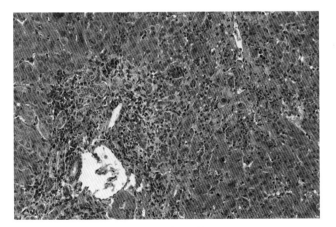

4.39 Drug-induced chronic active hepatitis.

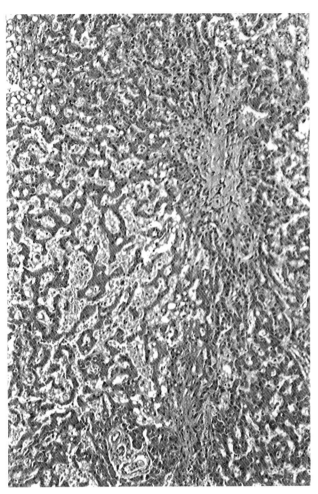

4.40 Drug-induced veno-occlusive disease.

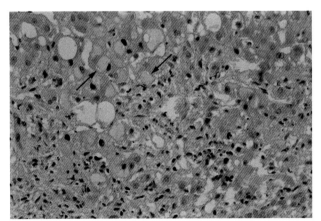

4.41 Disulfiram-induced liver injury.

4.42 Traumatic injury to liver

There is extensive irregular laceration of the liver which proved fatal. Many severe cases such as this are the result of road traffic accidents. The abdominal wall often remains intact.

4.43 Traumatic injury to liver

There is a small laceration filled with fibrin while some adjacent hepatocytes are necrotic. There is acute inflammatory cell infiltration. The biopsy was obtained during laparotomy several hours after the injury was sustained. Apart from the frankly necrotic liver tissue at the site of the injury, other areas at some distance from the main lesion may show centrilobular zonal degeneration or necrosis which is presumably ischemic in nature. Cholestasis also may supervene as a manifestation of shock. × 117 Hematoxylin and eosin.

4.44 Irradiation injury to liver

The upper and outer aspect of the liver has a mottled appearance due to necrosis induced by X-irradiation applied to the chest wall in the treatment of carcinoma of the breast. Modern methods of radiotherapy do not produce such injuries. Irradiation may cause also more generalized centrilobular degeneration and necrosis of hepatocytes with obliteration of central veins similar to that seen in veno-occlusive disease.

4.45 Anthracosis involving liver

Carbon pigment within macrophages situated in the subserous lymphatic network of the liver gives the surface of the organ a mottled appearance. Pigmentation is less obvious on naked-eye examination of cut surfaces but carbon-laden macrophages may be present in portal tracts. This liver is from a coal miner dying of anthraco-silicosis.

4.46 Granulomatous hepatitis induced by foreign material

Granulomas with a foreign body giant-cell reaction may be seen in liver biopsies, especially from drug addicts. They are, presumably, a reaction to binding material in the drug preparation given by intravenous injection. The lesions are found usually in portal tracts. There may be histological evidence also of virus B hepatitis transmitted parenterally, or there may be, as in this case, a less specific chronic inflammatory change throughout the liver, the pathogenesis of which is uncertain. × 146 Hematoxylin and eosin.

4.47 Mineral oil granuloma

The expanded portal tract contains numerous droplets of oil. The two largest in the centre of the field have induced a foreign body reaction with macrophages at their margins. This oil was derived from liquid paraffin which the patient ingested in large amounts over a period of many months. A similar reaction may be induced by oil absorbed into the portal circulation from rectal suppositories. × 187 Martius-scarlet-blue.

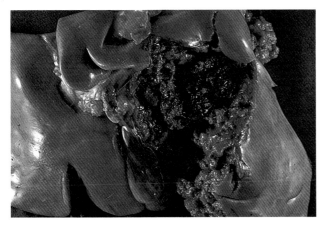

4.42 Traumatic injury to liver.

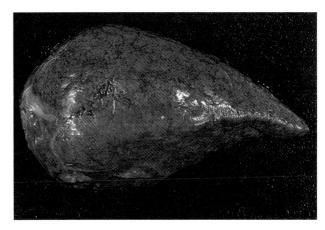

4.45 Anthracosis involving liver.

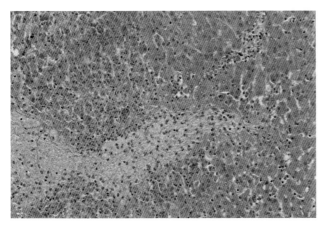

4.43 Traumatic injury to liver.

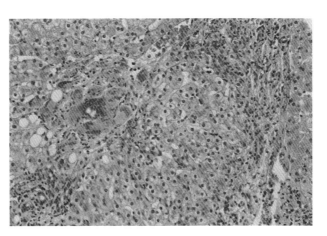

4.46 Granulomatous hepatitis induced by foreign material.

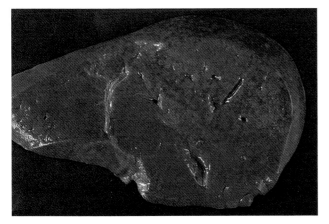

4.44 Irradiation injury to liver.

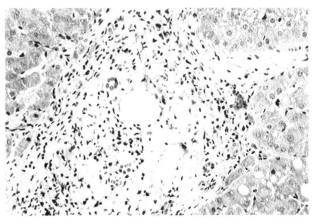

4.47 Mineral oil granuloma.

CHAPTER 5

Alcoholic and Nutritional Disorders

The two topics of alcoholic and nutritional disorders are included in one chapter because they share certain pathological features. It does not imply that malnutrition is an essential factor in the pathogenesis of alcoholic liver disease.

5.1 Alcoholic fatty liver

This biopsy shows extensive large-droplet fatty change but no necrosis and no hepatitis. There is an irregular distribution of small groups of parenchymal cells with relatively little steatosis; and in less severe cases of alcoholic fatty liver the position of fat-laden hepatocytes in the liver lobules remains haphazard, with no distinctive zonal pattern. There is often little clinical evidence of liver disease in such cases apart from hepatomegaly. × 45 Hematoxylin and eosin.

5.2 Alcoholic fatty liver: fat cyst formation

The majority of fat droplets are large and displace nuclei to their cell margins. In the centre of the field fat cysts have formed by fusion of adjacent droplets following loss of attenuated hepatocyte cytoplasm. This fat will undergo phagocytosis by macrophages, but it is possible that some may enter vascular channels and become a source of small fat emboli. Fat cysts may occur in severe hepatic steatosis from any cause. × 75 Hematoxylin and eosin.

5.3 Alcoholic fatty liver: fat granuloma

In the centre of the field immediately to the right of an hepatic venule is a small collection of macrophages which are vacuolated because of ingested lipid derived from fat cysts. Larger lesions which arise through coalescence of small granulomas can be responsible eventually for minor degrees of scarring unrelated to true alcoholic hepatitis. × 234 Hematoxylin and eosin.

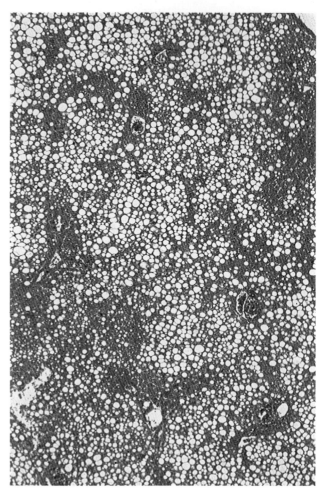

5.1 Alcoholic fatty liver.

5.4 Alcoholic fatty liver: centrilobular fibrosis

This is a case of alcoholic fatty liver without hepatitis. The blue connective tissue stain shows some thickening of the centrilobular vein and fibrosis extending into adjacent parenchyma. This lesion is seen in a minority of alcoholics with fatty liver and may be a precursor of central hyaline sclerosis (**5.22**). As in experimental alcoholic liver disease in primates it would appear that the fibrotic process can develop in the absence of inflammation or severe hepatocyte damage. × 146 Martius-scarlet-blue.

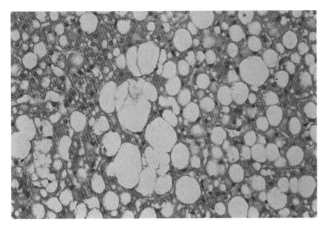

5.2 Alcoholic fatty liver: fat cyst formation.

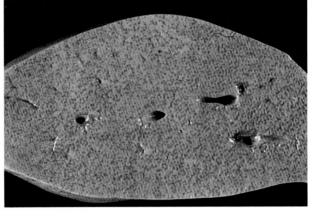

5.5 Alcoholic fatty liver and necrosis.

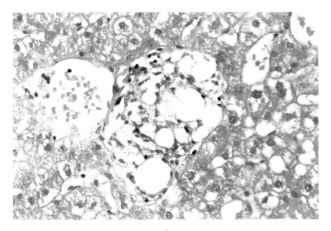

5.3 Alcoholic fatty liver: fat granuloma.

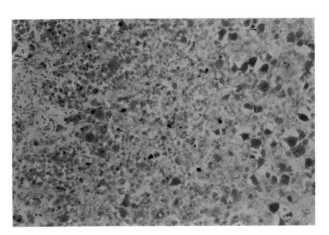

5.6 Alcoholic fatty liver and necrosis.

5.5 Alcoholic fatty liver and necrosis

This patient died of liver failure following an episode of excessive drinking. The liver is pale because of fatty change but this is less severe in the darker centrilobular zones which have undergone necrosis. Centrilobular zonal necrosis from alcohol or other causes (**4.16**) imparts a fine mottled appearance to the cut surface of the liver.

5.6 Alcoholic fatty liver and necrosis

The centrilobular zone in the centre of the field is necrotic and shows cholestasis. Fatty change is evident peripherally. This specimen also is from a case of fatal liver failure which followed a severe bout of drinking. While alcohol can be responsible directly for hepatocyte damage, this is probably aggravated in such cases by hypoglycemic shock with circulatory failure. × 117 Sudan IV and hematoxylin.

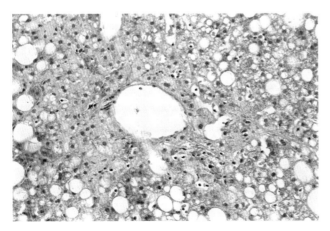

5.4 Alcoholic fatty liver: centrilobular fibrosis.

5.7 Alcoholic fatty liver and mild hepatitis

There is extensive fatty change, the majority of hepatocytes containing large fat droplets with marginal displacement of cell nuclei. There is mild chronic inflammation with fibrosis in the portal tracts. A centrilobular vein is seen (centre right), and in comparison with the biopsy shown in **5.4** there is no centrilobular fibrosis. Nor is there any evidence of important hepatocyte damage such as hyaline or hydropic degeneration. Alcohol withdrawal would probably lead to the return of a normal pattern of liver histology at this stage of the disease. × 75 Hematoxylin and eosin.

5.8 Alcoholic hepatitis

This shows the cut surface of a liver which was of rather firm consistency. There are tiny islands of parenchyma which are pale because of fatty change; they are separated by greyer areas which were seen on histological examination to consist of collagen and an inflammatory cell infiltrate. The faint green discoloration is due to intrahepatic cholestasis. Although there is no evidence of established alcoholic cirrhosis (cf. **5.28**, **5.29**), nevertheless, there may be a fatal outcome at this stage of the disease because of either extensive liver cell damage or diffuse fibrosis with portal hypertension.

5.9 Alcoholic hepatitis

The cardinal histological features of this disease are: (a) fatty change; (b) hydropic degeneration of hepatocytes (small arrows); (c) Mallory bodies—hyaline bodies in hepatocyte cytoplasm (large arrows); (d) diffuse fibrosis; (e) inflammatory cell infiltration including polymorphs. All these features are present here. × 146 Hematoxylin and eosin.

5.10 Alcoholic hepatitis

Notice the prominence of the connective tissue stroma which is stained red, especially in the central part of the lobule (central vein, bottom left). Fibrous thickening of sinusoidal walls is a common feature of established alcoholic liver disease and need not be preceded by evidence of active hepatitis (**5.4**). Fatty change is mild in this case, but this is not uncommon when alcoholism has persisted for prolonged periods. The portal area on the right is mildly infiltrated with acute and chronic inflammatory cells. The presence of neutrophil polymorphs and diffuse fibrosis, as illustrated in the biopsy, always suggests that such a case of chronic hepatitis is due to alcohol. × 117 Van Gieson's stain and hematoxylin.

5.11 Alcoholic hepatitis: forms of hepatocyte damage

This section shows various indications of liver cell damage attributed to prolonged alcohol intake. The most characteristic is hyaline degeneration of cytoplasm manifest as dense eosinophilic bodies (Mallory bodies) some of which are indicated by small arrows. Some other hepatocytes show hydropic swelling (ballooning degeneration) and there are a few small foci of acidophilic degeneration (large arrows). These latter features may be seen in other types of liver injury, e.g. viral hepatitis. There is a mild diffuse inflammatory cell infiltration including neutrophil polymorphs. It must be noted, however, that all these features may be found occasionally in hepatitis from causes other than alcohol (e.g. **5.32**). × 187 Hematoxylin and eosin.

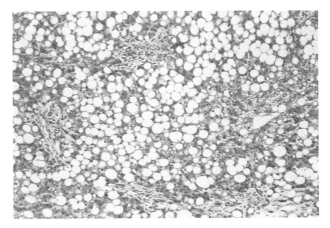

5.7 Alcoholic fatty liver and mild hepatitis.

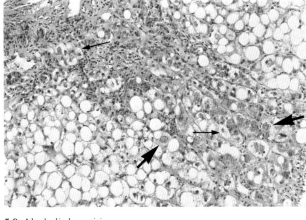

5.9 Alcoholic hepatitis.

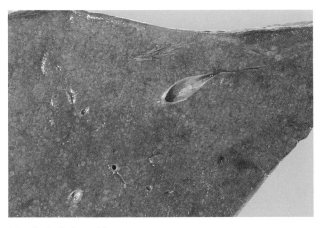

5.8 Alcoholic hepatitis.

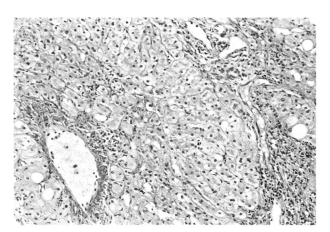

5.10 Alcoholic hepatitis.

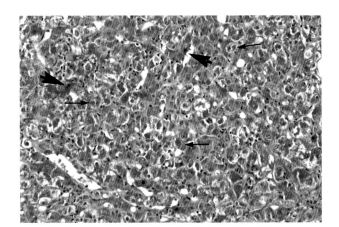

5.11 Alcoholic hepatitis: forms of hepatocyte damage.

5.12 Alcoholic hepatitis: hyaline degeneration of hepatocytes

Sections stained by Mallory's method or its various trichrome modifications usually but not invariably demonstrate acidophilic staining of hyaline material. The many Mallory bodies in this field, especially top right, can be identified therefore by their red colour. However, in a minority of cases the bodies are, apparently, basophilic and are shown faintly by the blue component of this stain mixture. × 220 Martius-scarlet-blue.

5.13 Alcoholic hepatitis: hyaline degeneration of hepatocytes

Nodular hyaline material is present in the cytoplasm of some hepatocytes. While staining deeply with eosin the edges are often ill-defined as are the boundaries of the affected cells. Many of the hepatocytes are probably damaged irreparably and some show clear evidence of necrosis with loss of nuclei. Cholestasis is also seen (arrow). × 234 Hematoxylin and eosin.

5.14 Alcoholic hepatitis: hyaline degeneration of hepatocytes

This section has been treated with an antibody to alcoholic hyalin using the immunoperoxidase method, and shows brown staining of Mallory bodies. The antibody is prepared to Mallory bodies which have been isolated from homogenates of alcohol-damaged liver. Because of its sensitivity and specificity, this method facilitates assessment of the severity and extent of hyaline degeneration. × 277 Immunoperoxidase.

5.15 Alcoholic hepatitis: hyaline degeneration of hepatocytes

In the centre of the field there is a necrotic hepatocyte with cytoplasmic hyalin and surrounded by a cuff of acute inflammatory cells. Large collections of neutrophil polymorphs may surround small groups of hepatocytes containing Mallory bodies. However, the phenomenon is seen with only a proportion of viable or necrotic hyaline hepatocytes. Where there are small discrete foci of neutrophils alone, serial sections usually demonstrate a close relationship to Mallory bodies. This feature is generally found in severe cases of alcoholic hepatitis. × 385 Hematoxylin and eosin.

5.16 Alcoholic hepatitis: hyaline degeneration of bile ductular epithelium

Occasionally in alcoholic hepatitis, hyaline degeneration may involve bile duct epithelium as well as hepatocytes. One example of this is shown here (arrow). × 300 Hematoxylin and eosin.

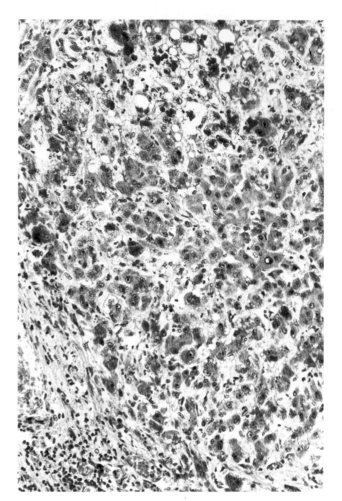

5.12 Alcoholic hepatitis: hyaline degeneration of hepatocytes.

5.17 Alcoholic hepatitis: giant mitochondria in hepatocytes

Giant mitochondria appear as circular or oval eosinophilic bodies within the hepatocyte cytoplasm. Some are almost as large as the cell nucleus (arrows). Unlike Mallory bodies their edges are always sharply defined. The larger specimens may be mistaken for erythrocytes. These large mitochondria are seen in certain cases of human alcoholic liver disease and may be induced in experimental animals fed alcohol over many weeks. They have been noted also in regenerating liver following partial hepatectomy. × 300 Hematoxylin and eosin.

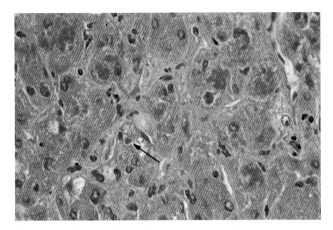

5.13 Alcoholic hepatitis: hyaline degeneration of hepatocytes.

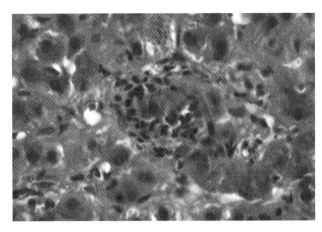

5.15 Alcoholic hepatitis: hyaline degeneration of hepatocytes.

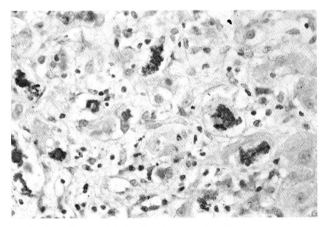

5.14 Alcoholic hepatitis: hyaline degeneration of hepatocytes.

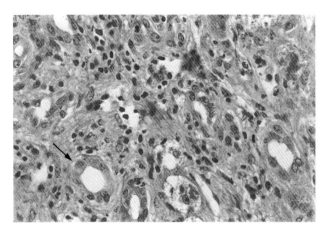

5.16 Alcoholic hepatitis: hyaline degeneration of bile ductular epithelium.

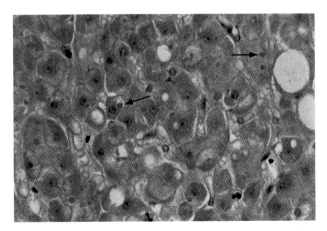

5.17 Alcoholic hepatitis: giant mitochondria in hepatocytes.

5.18 Alcoholic hepatitis: ballooning degeneration of hepatocytes

Although ballooning (hydropic) degeneration of hepatocytes is more commonly associated with viral hepatitis it may be seen in cases of alcoholic liver damage in addition to fatty change and hyaline degeneration. Ballooned cells are unusually numerous in this case, especially in the centre of the field. There are many more peripherally situated hepatocytes, especially above and to the left of centre, which contain large fat droplets and so resemble ballooned cells on account of swelling and apparently empty cytoplasm. The ballooned cells, however, retain centrally placed nuclei which are smaller than normal. While alcoholic and viral hepatitis may co-exist, there was no evidence for such an association in this case. × 113 Hematoxylin and eosin.

5.19 Alcoholic hepatitis: intrahepatic cholestasis

As in other forms of chronic hepatitis, intrahepatic cholestasis may be prominent. In this field, in addition to fatty change, hepatitis and fibrosis there are several dark, almost black, plugs of bile in distended bile capillaries (arrows). These patients usually suffer from a cholestatic type of jaundice. The variable incidence of cholestasis in alcoholic liver disease cannot be explained readily, although there may be an element of biliary obstruction in some cases related to alcoholic pancreatitis. Some patients with alcoholic hepatitis and pancreatitis also suffer from hemolytic anemia (Zieve's syndrome), and it is conceivable that the damaged liver may be unable to cope with the excretion of additional bilirubin derived from excessive blood destruction. While cholestasis is found generally in the more severe cases of alcoholic liver damage, it has been noted rarely in alcoholic fatty liver without hepatitis. × 117 Hematoxylin and eosin.

5.20 Alcoholic hepatitis: hemosiderin in liver

Granules of hemosiderin pigment are found in hepatocytes in some cases of alcoholism. The cells most affected are adjacent to portal tracts. All degrees of severity are encountered up to a condition similar to hemochromatosis; indeed alcoholism has been regarded as a cause of hemochromatosis (**9.1, 9.4, 9.9**). The example illustrated here is much less severe than this, with no involvement of bile duct epithelium or encrustation of iron pigment on collagen. Some alcoholic beverages such as red wine are rich in iron but the phenomenon cannot always be explained simply by excessive intake of iron in combination with alcohol. It is reported that alcohol causes increased absorption of iron. It is possible that hemosiderin in the liver contributes to the development of fibrosis and cirrhosis, but it is by no means essential for this. × 117 Perls' stain for hemosiderin.

5.21 Alcoholic hepatitis: chronic active hepatitis

The upper left portion of this field shows a chronic inflammatory process spreading into the parenchyma with destruction of adjacent hepatocytes (piecemeal necrosis). The biopsy is from a chronic alcoholic, and while the liver is not fatty, a few Mallory bodies are present (arrows). Only a minority of cases of alcoholic liver disease show prominent piecemeal necrosis which is evidence of chronic active hepatitis. The pathogenesis of such cases is uncertain as it is seldom possible to establish the co-existence of an additional liver-damaging agent such as viral infection or hepatotoxic drug. × 187 Hematoxylin and eosin.

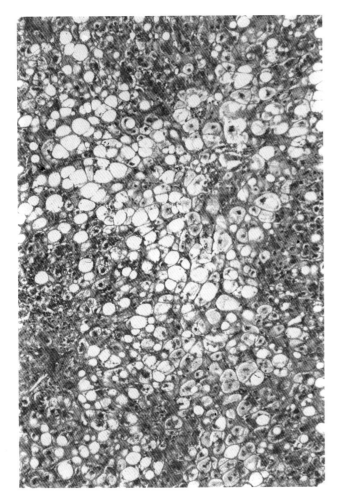

5.18 Alcoholic hepatitis: ballooning degeneration of hepatocytes.

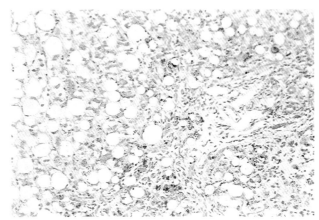

5.20 Alcoholic hepatitis: hemosiderin in liver.

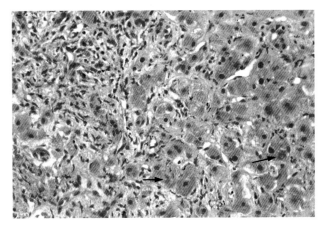

5.21 Alcoholic hepatitis: chronic active hepatitis.

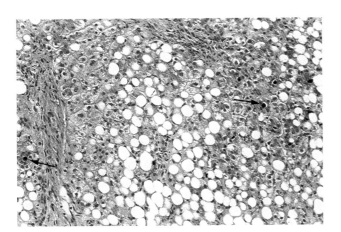

5.19 Alcoholic hepatitis: intrahepatic cholestasis.

5.22 Alcoholic hepatitis: central hyaline necrosis and sclerosis

The central part of the liver lobule is shown above. There is extensive hydropic and hyaline degeneration with necrosis of hepatocytes in this zone. The centrilobular vein has disappeared, having been obliterated by fibrous tissue. This is a severe form of alcoholic liver damage with a high mortality rate. There is little or no attempt at regeneration of surviving parenchyma but, despite the absence of cirrhosis, portal hypertension occurs because of occlusion of hepatic venules. ×117 Hematoxylin and eosin.

5.23 Alcoholic hepatitis: central hyaline sclerosis

A portal tract is seen on the left and a centrilobular zone on the right. The latter is occupied by scar tissue which replaces hepatocytes and the centrilobular vein. ×117 Martius-scarlet-blue.

5.24 Alcoholic hepatitis: extensive hepatic sclerosis

There is extensive sclerosis, much of the liver consisting of fibrous tissue which is stained blue. There is little or no nodular regeneration of surviving parenchyma to justify a diagnosis of cirrhosis. Diffuse fibrosis such as this is a characteristic feature of many cases of severe alcoholic liver damage. ×79 Martius-scarlet-blue.

5.25 Alcoholic hepatitis: extensive hepatic sclerosis

Part of the liver of a chronic alcoholic who died from massive esophageal hemorrhage. It was of firm leathery consistency and very difficult to cut. Much of the cut surface has a smooth pale yellow-grey appearance where the parenchyma has been replaced almost entirely by collagen. The cuff of necrosis around the hepatic vein may be attributed to posthemorrhagic shock as there was no gross vascular occlusion.

5.26 Alcoholic hepatitis: intrahepatic venous occlusion

The lumen of the hepatic venous radicle is narrowed because of subendothelial proliferation of connective tissue, an appearance similar to that seen in veno-occlusive disease (**3.20**). It is very unusual in alcoholic liver disease and may be caused by ingestion of toxic substances in addition to ethanol. There is also extensive fibrosis and small nodules of surviving parenchyma. ×71 Masson's trichrome stain.

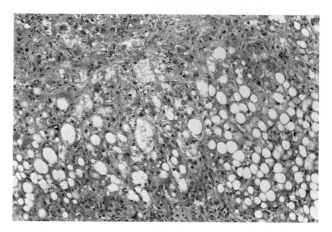

5.22 Alcoholic hepatitis: central hyaline necrosis and sclerosis.

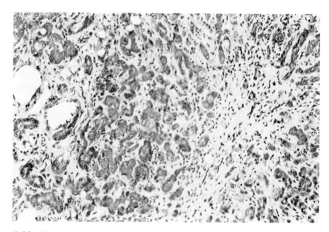

5.23 Alcoholic hepatitis: central hyaline sclerosis.

5.27 Alcoholic hepatitis: intrahepatic venous occlusion

A higher magnification showing considerable narrowing of the lumen of the intrahepatic vein by loose subintimal connective tissue. There is no evidence of thrombosis. ×117 Masson's trichrome stain.

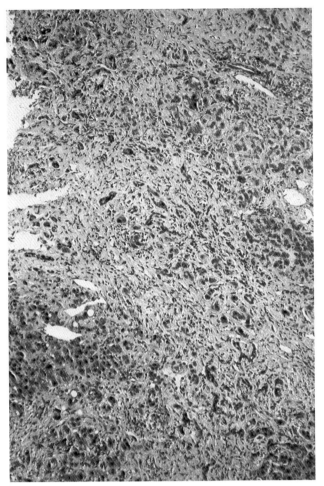

5.24 Alcoholic hepatitis: extensive hepatic sclerosis.

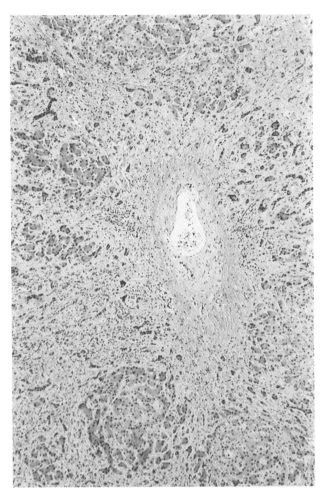

5.26 Alcoholic hepatitis: intrahepatic venous occlusion.

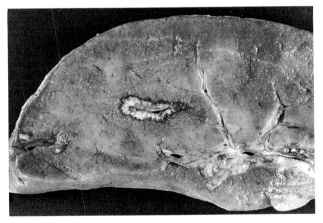

5.25 Alcoholic hepatitis: extensive hepatic sclerosis.

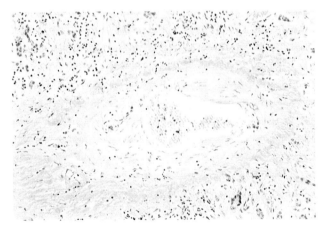

5.27 Alcoholic hepatitis: intrahepatic venous occlusion.

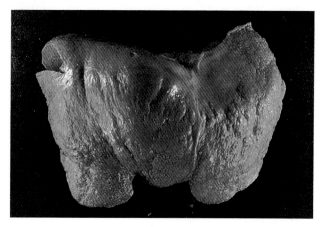

5.28 Alcoholic cirrhosis.

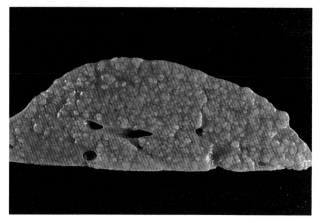

5.29 Alcoholic cirrhosis.

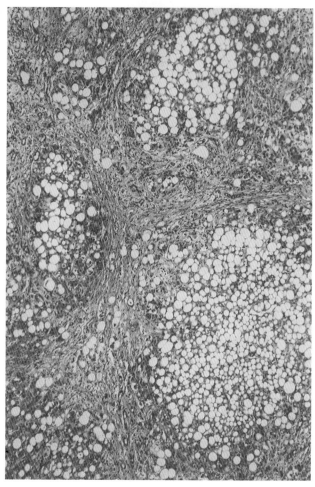

5.30 Alcoholic cirrhosis (early).

5.28 Alcoholic cirrhosis

The liver is pale due to fatty change and presents a fine granular surface. At this early stage of micronodular cirrhosis the organ is usually larger than normal.

5.29 Alcoholic cirrhosis

The nodules are fatty and separated by depressed bands of fibrous tissue. While of a larger size than in the specimen illustrated in **5.28**, they are relatively small compared to those in typical post-hepatitis (macronodular) cirrhosis (**6.20**). The term 'indeterminate cirrhosis' is used in such cases.

5.30 Alcoholic cirrhosis (early)

The parenchyma consists of small islands of fatty liver separated by broad bands of fibrous tissue which is infiltrated with inflammatory cells and contains proliferated bile ductules. Fatty change is less prominent in many cases of similar chronicity. × 71 Hematoxylin and eosin.

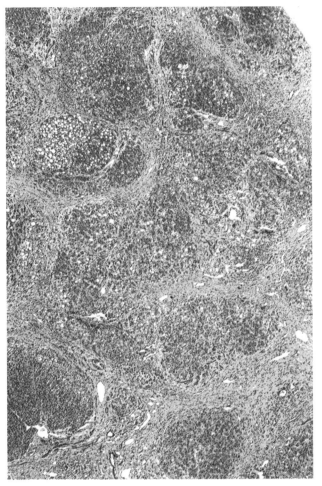

5.31 Alcoholic cirrhosis.

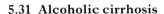

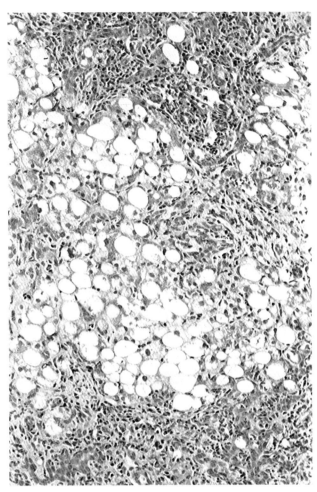

5.32 Severe liver injury complicating jejuno-ileal anastomosis for obesity.

5.31 Alcoholic cirrhosis

This is a fairly typical case, the hepatic parenchyma consisting of small nodules separated by fibrous tissue which is stained green. Note the small size of these nodules, the majority being no larger than liver lobules or parts of lobules. Unlike coarse macronodular cirrhosis the nodules contain no discrete vessels or diminutive portal tracts. ×45 Masson's trichrome stain.

5.32 Severe liver injury complicating jejuno-ileal anastomosis for obesity

Some cases develop very severe and even fatal liver disease although re-establishment of the normal intestinal anatomy may prevent such an outcome. Liver biopsy shows features which can be identical to severe alcoholic liver injury. In this example there is fatty and hydropic degeneration of hepatocytes together with extensive chronic inflammatory changes. Other conditions with histopathological features which can mimic alcoholic hepatitis include certain cases of chronic inflammatory bowel disease, chronic pancreatitis, chronic methotrexate poisoning, and some metabolic disorders such as Wilson's disease and abetalipoproteinemia. ×113 Hematoxylin and eosin.

5.33 Liver in obesity

Conspicuous fatty change may be found in the livers of obese subjects without significant liver dysfunction, and of similar severity to that seen in alcoholism (**5.1**). When less severe the distribution of fat varies; usually it is of the large-droplet type and is most marked in the centrilobular zones, as in this case. Small portal tracts can be identified at the right edge and bottom of the illustration, surrounded by apparently normal parenchyma. It is possible that these cases have increased susceptibility to various liver-damaging agents and minor degrees of portal and focal inflammation sometimes co-exist with the fatty change. The severe hepatitis in obese subjects subjected to jejuno-ileal anastomosis (**5.32**) may develop from these minor lesions. × 71 Hematoxylin and eosin.

5.34 Liver in obesity

In addition to steatosis there are several tiny foci of inflammation possibly related to ruptured fat cysts. Some portal tracts (not seen) were infiltrated by lymphocytes. × 117 Hematoxylin and eosin.

5.35 Kwashiorkor

The liver in this fatal case shows severe large-droplet fatty change and some malaria pigment in Kupffer cells (**8.20**). These patients do not have clinical evidence of significant liver dysfunction apart from hypoproteinemia. Hepatitis and fibrosis are mild or absent and cirrhosis does not ensue. The degree of fatty change is variable and in less severe cases tends to be periportal in distribution. Its severity may depend on the quality of carbohydrate in the protein-deficient diet, being aggravated by excessive intake of sucrose rather than starch. Death is often associated with the development of immune deficiency and increased susceptibility to various infections. × 75 Hematoxylin and eosin.

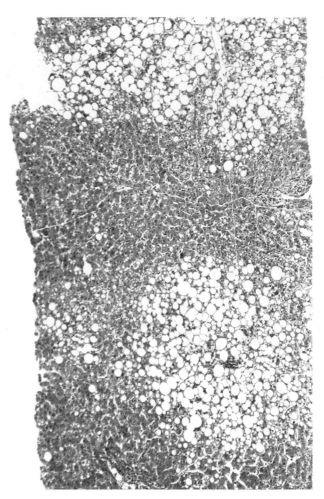

5.33 Liver in obesity.

5.36 Liver in infantile gastroenteritis

In this liver which had been fixed in a solution of osmium tetroxide, fat is shown by its black colour. It is most prominent in periportal hepatocytes. Hepatic steatosis is often prominent in infants infected with pathogenic strains of *E. coli*, but there is usually no clinical evidence of liver disorder. Fatty liver can develop quickly in this and other acute illnesses associated with severe vomiting with or without diarrhea. It resolves over a period of weeks after recovery. Cases of infantile marasmus do not have fatty liver or other evidence of liver damage; however, there may be hepatocyte atrophy with shrinkage of liver cell plates. × 35 Osmium and safranin.

5.37 Liver damage associated with parenteral feeding

Severe cholestatic jaundice may occur in neonates fed parenterally for a variety of reasons, and the liver shows evidence of bile capillary cholestasis. The author has had experience of a similar phenomenon in older patients. This illustration shows the liver biopsy from an adolescent fed parenterally for several months following small intestinal resection. There is centrilobular cholestasis (right) together with portal inflammation and hydropic degeneration of hepatocytes (left). A liver biopsy from this patient just before the onset of parenteral therapy was normal. The pathogenesis is not known. × 117 Hematoxylin and eosin.

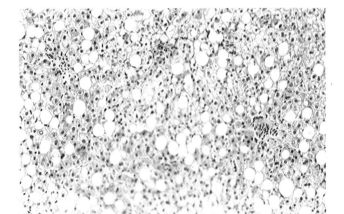

5.34 Liver in obesity.

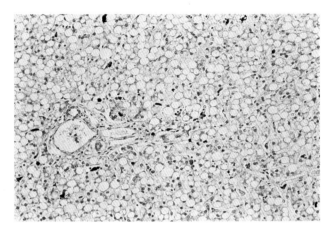

5.35 Kwashiorkor.

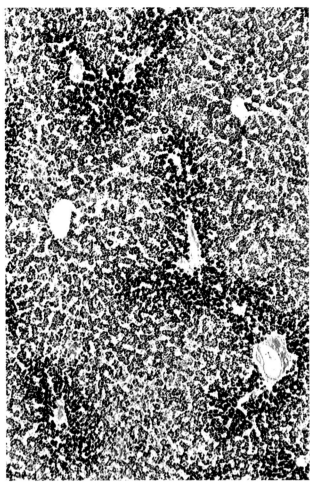

5.36 Liver in infantile gastroenteritis.

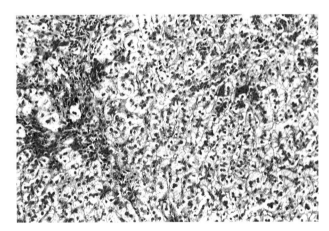

5.37 Liver damage associated with parenteral feeding.

CHAPTER 6

Viral Infections

6.1 Acute viral hepatitis

The appearances in this typical uncomplicated case include pleomorphism of hepatocytes, loss of a few hepatocytes (spotty necrosis) especially in a centrilobular zone (arrow), and inflammatory cell infiltration which is predominantly lymphocytic and conspicuous in the portal and periportal areas. There is no fatty change. These features occur diffusely throughout the liver and are similar for virus A, virus B and virus non-A non-B infections. × 47 Hematoxylin and eosin.

6.2 Acute viral hepatitis: lobular disarray

The orderly arrangement of hepatocytes is lost. A few individual cells are necrotic, with karyolysis, and there are other small foci of spotty necrosis or cell dropout where dead cells have been removed by phagocytes (arrows). Some surviving hepatocytes are enlarged and binucleate, a possible sign of regenerative activity. The cytoplasm of hepatocytes is eosinophilic and contains granules of lipofuscin and bile. Kupffer cells are prominent and there is infiltration of the lobules with inflammatory cells, mainly lymphocytes and histiocytes. Polymorphonuclear leukocytes and plasma cells are inconspicuous. × 234 Hematoxylin and eosin.

6.3 Acute viral hepatitis: ballooning (hydropic) degeneration of hepatocytes

This form of degeneration affects many hepatocytes in this field. These cells are swollen and their cytoplasm appears non-existent apart from a few granules and wisps of material adjacent to the nucleus. The change is related to dilatation of cisternae of the endoplasmic reticulum. Ballooned cells are frequent in viral hepatitis and probably responsible for much liver dysfunction in that disease. A similar type of degeneration may be seen in liver injury from other causes. While some affected cells undergo lysis, it is possible that others can recover. × 117 Hematoxylin and eosin.

6.4 Acute viral hepatitis: acidophilic degeneration and necrosis of hepatocytes

Several hepatocytes in this field are shrunken with intensely eosinophilic cytoplasm and small pyknotic nuclei. One necrotic cell of this type (Councilman body—arrow) has been extruded into a sinusoid where it would be ingested by phagocytes. Acidophilic cells, like ballooned cells, are not diagnostic of but are frequently found in viral hepatitis. They may persist for many weeks during the recovery phase. Being relatively small in number they probably contribute much less to liver dysfunction compared with ballooned cells. × 234 Hematoxylin and eosin.

6.5 Acute viral hepatitis: hepatocyte regeneration

Mitotic activity of hepatocytes and binucleate forms can be conspicuous even during the acute phase of the illness. In this field two hepatocytes (arrows) are in mitosis and many others show hydropic degeneration. There is infiltration with chronic inflammatory cells. × 300 Hematoxylin and eosin.

6.6 Acute viral hepatitis: stromal increase

While fibrosis is not apparent in conventional hematoxylin and eosin preparations of liver biopsies taken during the acute phase of the illness, connective tissue stains often demonstrate some stromal increase in portal and centrilobular zones. In this field fine red collagen fibres radiate out from centrilobular zones (arrows). This fibrotic process can undergo resolution and does not necessarily indicate unusual severity of the acute lesion or a tendency to chronicity. × 47 Van Gieson's stain and hematoxylin.

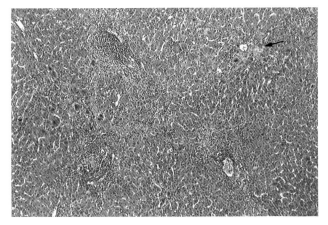

6.1 Acute viral hepatitis.

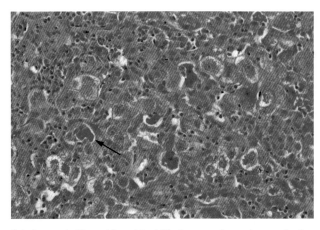

6.4 Acute viral hepatitis: acidophilic degeneration and necrosis of hepatocytes.

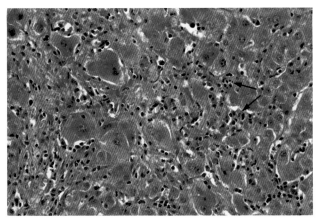

6.2 Acute viral hepatitis: lobular disarray.

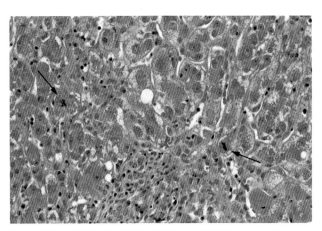

6.5 Acute viral hepatitis: hepatocyte regeneration.

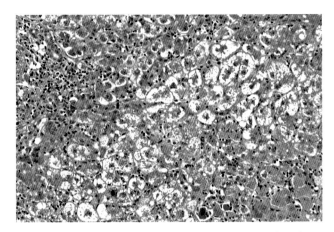

6.3 Acute viral hepatitis: ballooning (hydropic) degeneration of hepatocytes.

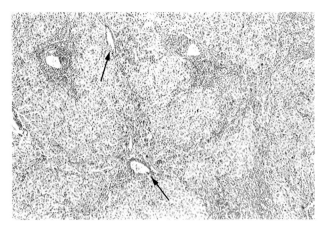

6.6 Acute viral hepatitis: stromal increase.

6.7 Acute fulminating hepatitis

The liver from a case of non-A non-B hepatitis dying within a week of the onset of symptoms. The organ was firm and swollen and shows areas of massive hemorrhagic necrosis which was confirmed by histological examination. When the patient survives into the second week the liver is generally pale, shrunken and soft ('acute yellow atrophy'), but is sometimes bile-stained. The nutmeg appearance of zonal and bridging necrosis may be seen in some fulminating cases.

6.8 Acute fulminating hepatitis

In this autopsy specimen there is confluent necrosis of liver parenchyma. All hepatocytes are necrotic with eosinophilic cytoplasm and pyknotic or karyolytic nuclei. The normal lobular pattern is retained, however, because of survival of mesenchymal tissue and portal tracts, and staining for reticulin would show retention of the connective tissue framework. The portal tracts contain viable proliferated bile ductules which stain deeply and there is also a mild inflammatory cell infiltrate which consists mainly of lymphocytes and macrophages. Sinusoids are rather congested especially in the centrilobular zone (centre). Necrosis appears to extend diffusely throughout the liver and sections taken from various sites had an identical appearance. × 71 Hematoxylin and eosin.

6.9 Acute hepatitis: survival after sub-massive necrosis

This patient lived for about 18 months after severe virus B hepatitis with sub-massive necrosis. Sufficient parenchyma remained to sustain life and become the foci of marked nodular regeneration resembling tumour deposits. Severe portal hypertension was responsible for several episodes of hematemesis. This probably aggravated the ischemic state of the cirrhotic nodules as much hepatic arterial and portal venous blood entering the liver passes through vessels in the fibrous septa which bypass the sinusoids of the nodules. Sectioning of the specimen showed clear evidence of necrosis in several nodules and some of these are illustrated in **3.29**. This would explain the terminal hepatic failure with encephalopathy in this case. Such cases of very coarse post-hepatitis cirrhosis, so-called 'subacute hepatitis', are unusual.

6.10 Subacute hepatitis

A case of severe virus B hepatitis who survived for several weeks. There is extensive loss of liver parenchyma with stromal condensation. This is prominent in the upper half of the illustration where there is heavy infiltration of condensed fibrous tissue by inflammatory cells, mostly lymphocytes. Bile ductular proliferation is also evident here. Below there are signs of early nodular regeneration in a surviving focus of liver parenchyma. There will be considerable distortion of the channels which drain bile from such nodules and this helps to explain the retention of bile pigment within bile capillaries which is evident here. × 62 Hematoxylin and eosin.

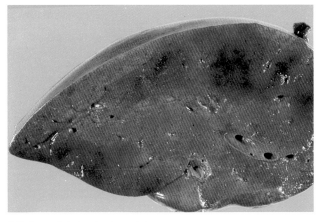

6.7 Acute fulminating hepatitis.

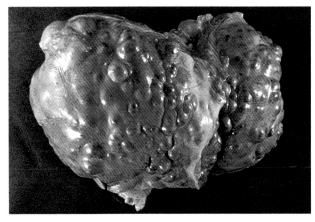

6.9 Acute hepatitis: survival after sub-massive necrosis.

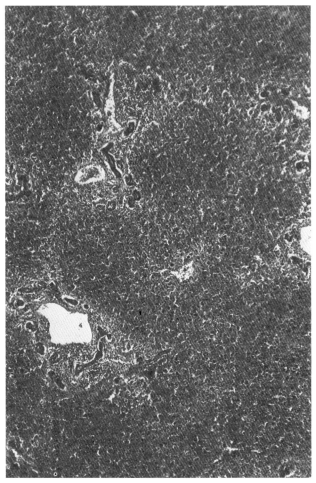

6.8 Acute fulminating hepatitis.

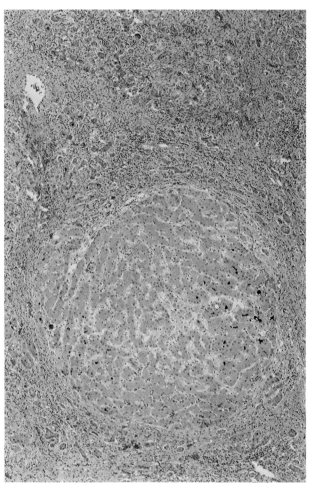

6.10 Subacute hepatitis.

6.11 Severe viral hepatitis: zonal necrosis

There is centrilobular necrosis of hepatocytes round hepatic venules (arrows). These lesions have a stellate pattern and further extension and fusion will establish bands of bridging necrosis (**6.12**). Centrilobular zonal necrosis and bridging necrosis are prominent in many post-mortem livers from cases of viral hepatitis. × 88 Hematoxylin and eosin.

6.12 Severe viral hepatitis: bridging necrosis

Bands of necrotic tissue of variable width connect adjacent centrilobular zones, or centrilobular zones and portal tracts. The portal area (top right) shows some inflammatory edema and irregularity of the limiting plate, but this does not amount to typical piecemeal necrosis as seen in chronic active hepatitis. The surviving parenchyma is unremarkable, but the degenerative and regenerative features already described (**6.1**, **6.5**) may also occur. Bile ductular proliferation and cholestasis are sometimes prominent. While bridging necrosis is certainly a sign of severe liver damage in viral hepatitis, it does not necessarily imply potential chronicity unless piecemeal necrosis and plasma-cell infiltration are prominent. × 47 Hematoxylin and eosin.

6.13 Severe viral hepatitis: pronounced lobular inflammation (lobular hepatitis)

There is marked infiltration of the liver lobules with inflammatory cells and the parenchyma shows the typical features of acute viral hepatitis. Lobular hepatitis also has been regarded as a sign of potential chronicity but in the absence of piecemeal necrosis complete resolution is possible. × 117 Hematoxylin and eosin.

6.14 Persistent viral hepatitis

The patient had mild symptoms and signs of liver dysfunction which were present for many months after the onset of the acute illness. There is now very little evidence of hepatocyte damage, the main feature being persistence of lymphocytic infiltration, especially in the portal tracts. In most cases this gradually resolves. × 71 Hematoxylin and eosin.

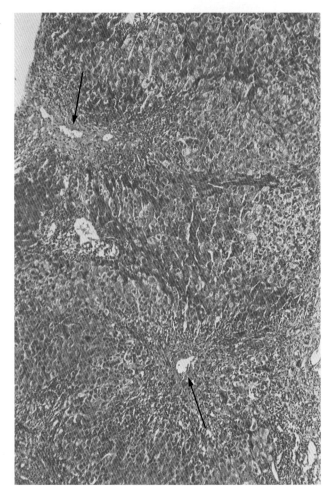

6.11 Severe viral hepatitis: zonal necrosis.

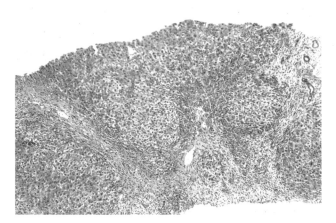

6.12 Severe viral hepatitis: bridging necrosis.

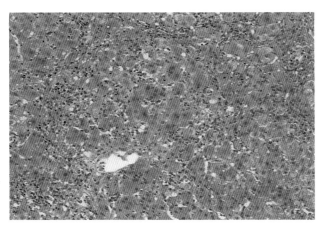

6.13 Severe viral hepatitis: pronounced lobular inflammation (lobular hepatitis).

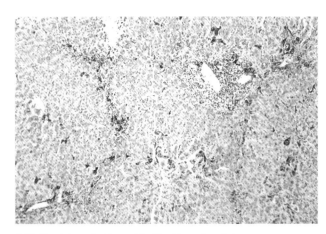

6.15 Persistent viral hepatitis: Kupffer cell activity.

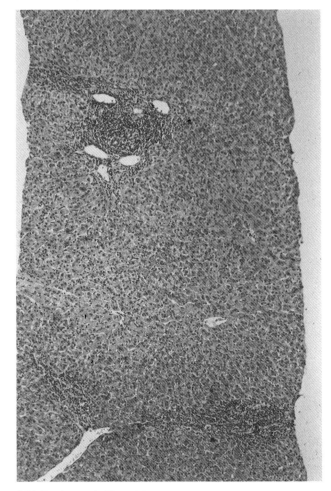

6.14 Persistent viral hepatitis.

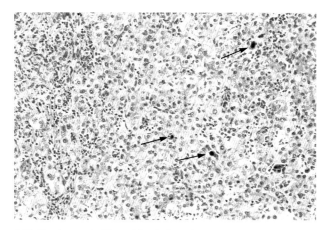

6.16 Persistent viral hepatitis: cholestasis.

minent by Prussian blue staining of ingested hemosiderin. In addition to this iron pigment, these cells may contain bile and periodic acid-Schiff positive material, all derived from ingested necrotic tissue. Hemosiderin is seen in Kupffer cells several weeks after the onset of acute viral hepatitis and can persist for months. × 54 Perls' method.

6.16 Persistent viral hepatitis: cholestasis

This specimen shows, in addition to the features of viral hepatitis, several dark bile thrombi (arrows) in bile capillaries. Such patients have a cholestatic type of jaundice which can persist for many months after the onset of the acute illness. Difficulty may be experienced in distinguishing this condition from cholangiohepatitis due to extrahepatic biliary obstruction (chapter 2), especially when neutrophil polymorphonuclear cell infiltration and bile ductular proliferation appear as additional histological features of these persistent viral infective cases. Cholestatic viral hepatitis will resolve eventually. × 117 Hematoxylin and eosin.

6.15 Persistent viral hepatitis: Kupffer cell activity

The specimen was taken during recovery from acute viral hepatitis. Many Kupffer cells are rendered pro-

6.17 Chronic active hepatitis from viral hepatitis

This patient gave a history of recurring attacks of hepatic insufficiency over a two-year period following fairly mild acute hepatitis, apparently a non-A non-B infection. Note the persistent portal and periportal inflammatory cell infiltration and irregular destruction (piecemeal necrosis) of adjacent hepatocytes (arrow). There is also a lobular lymphocytic infiltration and some hydropic swelling of other hepatocytes. Assessment of the prognosis of a case such as this can be difficult but the relatively long illness, type of infection, and piecemeal loss of hepatocytes are suggestive of chronic active hepatitis which can lead to cirrhosis. × 71 Hematoxylin and eosin.

6.18 Chronic active hepatitis from viral hepatitis

Another field from the case illustrated in **6.17** showing more clearly the piecemeal loss of hepatocytes, small islands of these cells surviving in the midst of the inflammatory cell infiltrate. The presence of plasma cells and fibroblast activity also favours the diagnosis of chronic active hepatitis. The assessment of prognosis in these cases is never easy and account must be taken also of the type of viral infection, post-hepatic cirrhosis being associated most frequently with non-A non-B infection and rarely, if ever, with A infection. × 187 Hematoxylin and eosin.

6.19 Chronic hepatitis from viral hepatitis

Chronicity is suggested in this case by the pronounced degree of portal and periportal lymphocytic infiltration and by nodular regenerative activity of parenchyma. Nevertheless subsequent biopsies showed remarkable regression of these features after one year and complete recovery by two years. × 71 Hematoxylin and eosin.

6.20 Posthepatitis cirrhosis

The liver has the typical pattern of macronodular cirrhosis, the parenchyma consisting of prominent nodules measuring up to 1 cm in diameter and separated by depressed fibrous septa. The etiology of such a lesion cannot be assessed from its gross appearance although it would be reasonable to exclude alcohol, hemochromatosis and primary biliary cirrhosis in this case.

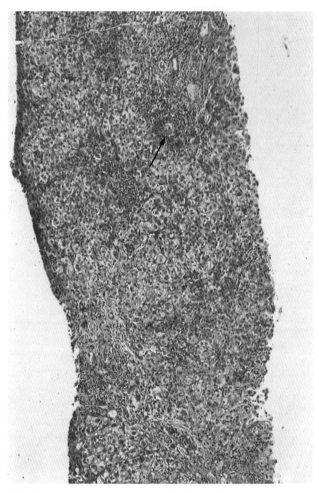

6.17 Chronic active hepatitis from viral hepatitis.

6.21 Posthepatitis cirrhosis

Much of the liver consists of large well-defined nodules separated by thin fibrous bands which link vascular structures. A few tiny venules are present within the nodules (arrow). On the right there is persistent chronic inflammatory activity and fibrosis with entrapped liver cells. The amount of this activity varies from case to case and in different parts of the same specimen. × 30 Van Gieson's stain and hematoxylin.

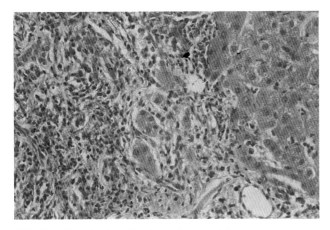

6.18 Chronic active hepatitis from viral hepatitis.

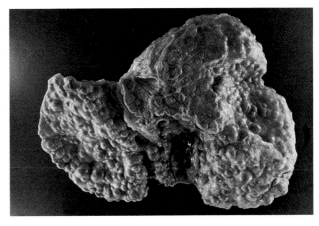

6.20 Posthepatitis cirrhosis.

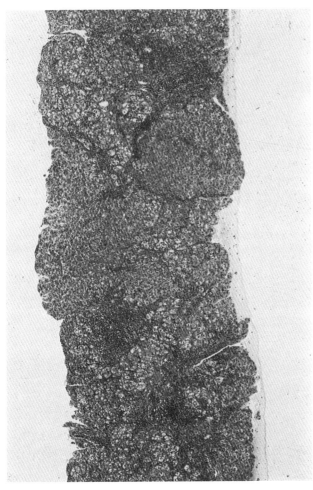

6.19 Chronic hepatitis from viral hepatitis.

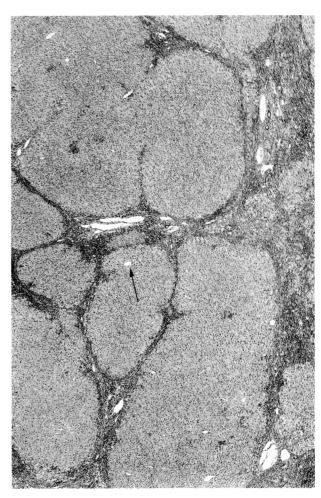

6.21 Posthepatitis cirrhosis.

6.22 Hepatitis B infection: ground-glass cells

The cytoplasm of some hepatocytes has a finely granular appearance like ground glass which contrasts with the much coarser granules seen in other hydropic cells. It is evident that ground-glass change need not involve the entire cell cytoplasm and that it may be separated from the margin of the cell by a narrow vacuolated rim. This is from a case of virus B infection with chronic active hepatitis. In such specimens the ground-glass hepatocytes are seen in clusters which have an irregular distribution in the liver. The appearance is attributable to hepatitis B virus surface antigen (HBsAg) in liver-cell cytoplasm. In electron microscopic preparations the antigen is seen as filamentous particles situated within the cisternae of proliferating and distorted agranular endoplasmic reticulum. × 300 Hematoxylin and eosin.

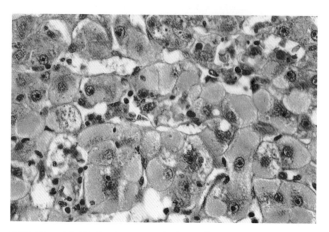

6.22 Hepatitis B infection: ground-glass cells.

6.23 Hepatitis B carrier: ground-glass cells

An aldehyde thionin-treated section shows dark blue staining of certain hepatocytes, which are ground-glass cells, in an otherwise normal liver. The patient was a symptomless carrier of the infection. The livers of immunosuppressed patients may also show HBsAg in the absence of an inflammatory reaction, but hepatitis can supervene with recovery of immune competence. × 283 Thionin.

6.24 HBsAg: orcein staining

A case of chronic active hepatitis in which hepatocytes containing HBsAg are stained brown by orcein. This stain also demonstrates elastic tissue in the walls of vessels (right). Positive staining of HBsAg may be achieved also with chromotrope aniline blue and aldehyde fuchsin, both of which impart a dark blue colour to the antigen. Neither is illustrated here. × 68 Orcein.

6.25 HBsAg: staining by the immunoperoxidase technique

The viral surface antigen is readily demonstrated in tissue sections treated with its antibody in the standard immunoperoxidase procedure. The dark brown positive reaction is confined to the cytoplasm of a cluster of infected hepatocytes and the absence of nuclear staining is also a prominent feature. Some liver cell plates (top left) are unstained and there are many inflammatory cells indicative of chronic hepatitis. × 117 Immunoperoxidase.

6.26 HBsAg: staining by the immunoperoxidase technique

A lower magnification of the specimen in **6.25** shows the irregular distribution of infected hepatocytes in a cirrhotic liver of macronodular type. This evidence of failure to eliminate the virus from the liver, which in most cases occurs during the acute phase of the illness, is often found in chronic hepatitis and cirrhosis complicating virus B infection. × 28 Immunoperoxidase.

6.27 HBsAg: staining by the immunoperoxidase technique

This immunoperoxidase-treated section shows many hepatocytes with marginal staining for HBsAg, a pattern which is associated particularly with persistent hepatitis and continuing hepatocyte destruction. Possibly in these cases of membranous staining the antigen is readily exposed to attack by activated lymphocytes which would lead to destruction of the infected hepatocytes. Of course other virus B antigens may be involved. × 187 Immunoperoxidase.

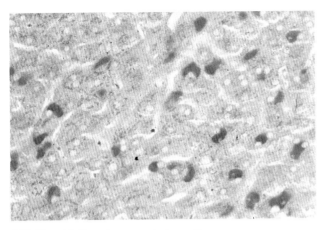

6.23 Hepatitis B carrier: ground-glass cells.

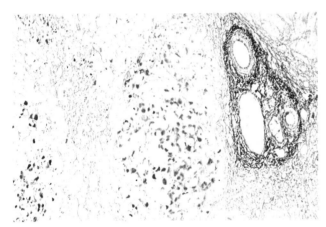

6.24 HBsAg: orcein staining.

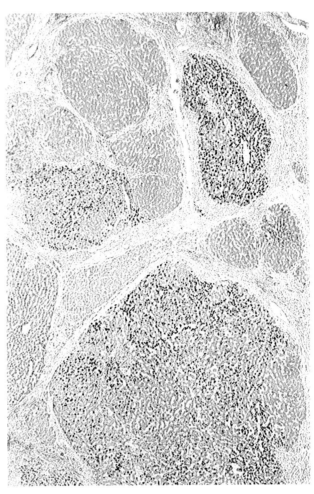

6.26 HBsAg: staining by the immunoperoxidase technique.

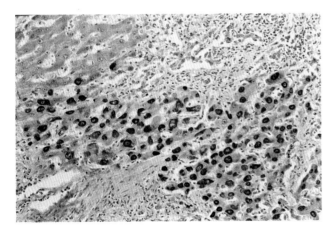

6.25 HBsAg: staining by the immunoperoxidase technique.

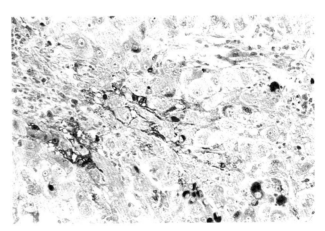

6.27 HBsAg: staining by the immunoperoxidase technique.

6.28 Herpes simplex hepatitis

A section from the liver of a young infant with fatal *Herpesvirus hominis* infection. There are numerous foci of coagulative necrosis, one of which is illustrated. The margin of the lesion is congested but there is little inflammatory response. At this low magnification it is evident that these are small discrete lesions which may just be visible to the naked eye (as small yellow spots) and that they have a haphazard distribution in the liver lobule. A similar disease occurs rarely in older children and adults as a consequence of immune deficiency. × 59 Hematoxylin and eosin.

6.29 Herpes simplex hepatitis

There was extensive hemorrhagic necrosis of this infant's liver. Of the few surviving viable hepatocytes which can be recognized in this field, some have intranuclear viral inclusions (arrows) which are rather basophilic, especially at their periphery. Some inclusions are surrounded by a halo which separates them from a rim of condensed nuclear chromatin. Extensive liver necrosis in this infection has been associated with infantile malnutrition. × 234 Hematoxylin and eosin.

6.30 Cytomegalovirus hepatitis

The liver of a three-month infant dying of an immune deficiency syndrome. The infected liver cells are swollen with basophilic cytoplasm, and contain central intranuclear inclusions with a peripheral halo which produces the characteristic 'owl's eye' appearance of this infection. Infected hepatocytes undergo necrosis leaving small foci of cell dropout in which inflammatory cells may collect. The number of these lesions varies from case to case. In some there is a notable inflammatory reaction to the infection which may be followed by fibrosis or take the form of granulomas with multinucleated giant cells. In younger babies there may be giant-cell transformation of hepatocytes. × 187 Hematoxylin and eosin.

6.31 Cytomegalovirus hepatitis

Another field from the case in **6.30** showing involvement of the epithelium of a bile ductule by virus (arrow). Vascular endothelial cells can be infected also. Infection of bile ductules may be responsible for cholestasis and cholangitis which may be seen in some cases. × 300 Hematoxylin and eosin.

6.32 Yellow fever

There is extensive parenchymal necrosis with survival of rims of hepatocytes round the central vein (lower right) and portal tract (left). This midzonal pattern of necrosis is characteristic of yellow fever. Liver cell degeneration and necrosis is of the acidophilic type and includes Kupffer cells. Many Kupffer cells survive however, and become prominent from ingestion of ceroid pigment and hemosiderin. Fatty change may be present also but is not seen in this field. There is some lymphocytic infiltration of the portal tracts. While death may be the result of liver parenchymal necrosis, many patients also suffer from extensive renal tubular damage. Those who recover have no persistent liver damage such as cholestasis, chronic hepatitis or cirrhosis. × 75 Hematoxylin and eosin.

6.33 Giant cell hepatitis

Post-mortem liver from a young infant with congenital rubella syndrome showing many enlarged multinucleated hepatocytes. In some there is cholestasis, but inflammatory cell infiltration is often inconspicuous, as in this case. For this reason the term 'giant cell transformation' is often more appropriate. Dissociation of giant cells from their neighbours is described, but in this case the hepatocyte separation is due probably to post-mortem autolysis. A variety of hepatic diseases in early infancy due to various infections, rhesus incompatibility, biliary atresia, inherited metabolic disorders etc., may be associated with similar giant cell transformation of hepatocytes. × 117 Hematoxylin and eosin.

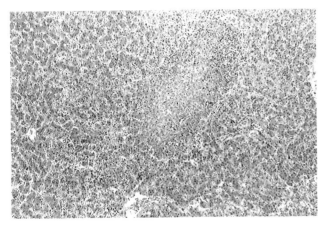

6.28 Herpes simplex hepatitis.

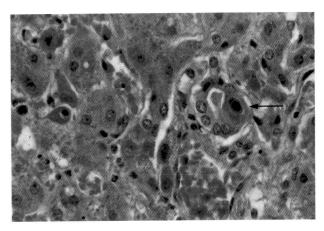

6.31 Cytomegalovirus hepatitis.

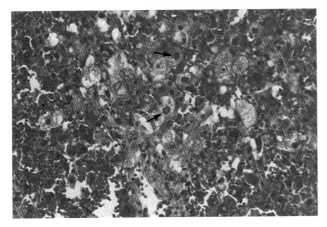

6.29 Herpes simplex hepatitis.

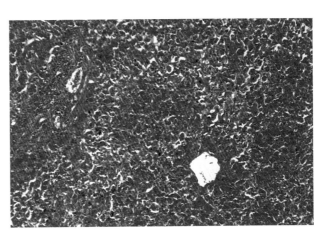

6.32 Yellow fever.

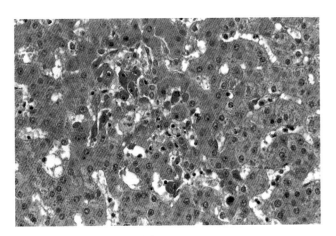

6.30 Cytomegalovirus hepatitis.

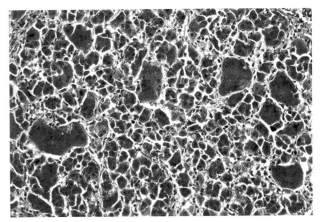

6.33 Giant cell hepatitis.

CHAPTER 7

Chronic Hepatitis

This chapter deals with those chronic inflammatory liver diseases of doubtful or unknown etiology which are not appropriate to other sections of the book.

7.1 Chronic active hepatitis

There is dense infiltration of portal tracts with chronic inflammatory cells. The tracts appear to be widened because of extension of this infiltrate into the surrounding periportal parenchyma, where there is destruction of hepatocytes (piecemeal necrosis). This imparts an irregular outline to the periphery of liver lobules. This biopsy is from a young woman with several years' history of progressive liver disease and with circulating smooth muscle antibody and anti-nuclear factor. An initial cause of liver injury such as viral hepatitis was not found. ×71 Hematoxylin and eosin.

7.2 Chronic active hepatitis

Another field from the biopsy illustrated in **7.1** shows more clearly the piecemeal destruction of hepatocytes in the periportal area where there is heavy infiltration with inflammatory cells, mainly lymphocytes. One hepatocyte shows acidophilic necrosis (small arrow). Regenerative activity is evident by widening of some liver cell plates and an indistinct rosette formation of hepatocytes (large arrow). Apart from piecemeal necrosis the severity of parenchymal damage varies from case to case; in some there are features similar to severe viral infection such as lobular hepatitis and bridging necrosis. ×187 Hematoxylin and eosin.

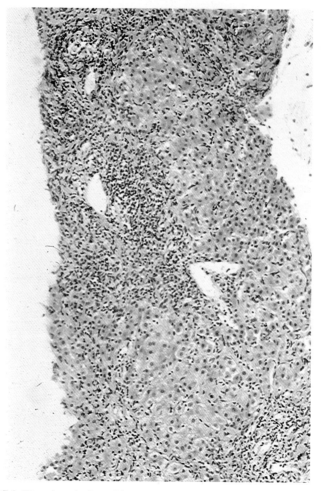

7.1 Chronic active hepatitis.

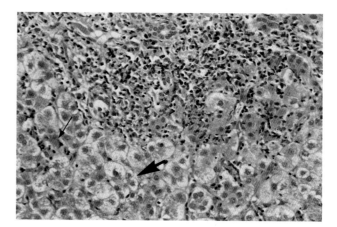

7.2 Chronic active hepatitis.

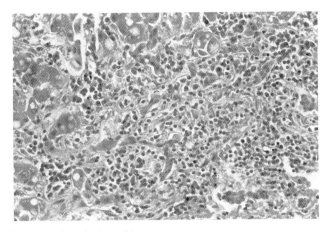

7.3 Chronic active hepatitis.

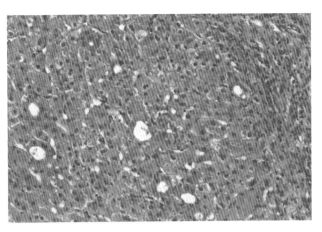

7.4 Chronic active hepatitis.

7.3 Chronic active hepatitis

Plasma cells are numerous in this periportal area where there is piecemeal necrosis. A few fibroblasts are present also. × 187 Hematoxylin and eosin.

7.4 Chronic active hepatitis

Hepatocyte regeneration with the formation of gland-like structures is conspicuous in this field. This feature should not be confused with bile duct proliferation which is not characteristic of chronic active hepatitis. × 158 Hematoxylin and eosin.

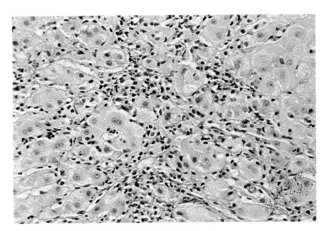

7.5 Chronic active hepatitis.

7.5 Chronic active hepatitis

A periportal area showing an increase in fine red-staining type III collagen fibres, the product of local fibroblast activity. In sections stained to show reticulin these fibres are argyrophilic. In cases surviving for several years, continuing fibrogenesis can lead to cirrhosis, with excessive amounts of coarser refractile type I collagen. × 187 Van Gieson's stain and hematoxylin.

7.6 Chronic active hepatitis progressing to cirrhosis

The cut surface of the liver of a young woman who suffered from chronic active hepatitis of unknown cause for a number of years. There are numerous small foci of nodular regeneration, some rather indistinct. With longer survival a macronodular type of cirrhosis would develop similar in appearance to post-viral hepatitic cirrhosis.

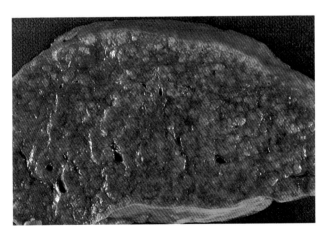

7.6 Chronic active hepatitis progressing to cirrhosis.

7.7 Chronic persistent hepatitis

As in chronic active hepatitis there is prominence and widening of the portal tracts with a chronic inflammatory cell infiltrate. While this may spill over into the adjacent liver parenchyma, piecemeal destruction of hepatocytes is absent or present to only a minor degree, as in this case. Lobular parenchymal damage is also less marked although there is some swelling of a few centrilobular hepatocytes. Chronic persistent hepatitis can remain static for many years and may resolve. Both the active and persistent varieties of chronic hepatitis may be initiated by various liver-damaging agents including viral infections and drugs, and these possibilities must be considered in the investigation of any case. It is customary to use the term 'chronic persistent hepatitis' for patients with no identifiable cause of liver injury and whose clinical illness has persisted for at least six months. × 71 Hematoxylin and eosin.

7.8 Non-specific reactive hepatitis

The histological features as seen in this field can be similar to chronic persistent hepatitis with mild or moderate lymphocytic infiltration of portal tracts. Small foci of cell dropout are recognized by collections of inflammatory cells in the parenchyma, and these may form indistinct granulomas. Kupffer cells are often prominent although this is not a striking feature of this case. Unlike chronic persistent hepatitis these changes are distributed less evenly throughout the liver, and may be seen in only a minority of multiple blocks taken from autopsy specimens. Accordingly there may be little or no clinical evidence of hepatic disorder, the illness often being some febrile infective condition or abdominal disease arising outwith the liver. Similar patchy lesions have been attributed to the ingestion of certain drugs (**4.33**). × 32 Hematoxylin and eosin.

7.9 Chronic septal hepatitis

This lesion may be regarded as a form of chronic persistent or non-specific reactive hepatitis in which portal inflammation and fibrosis extend into the parenchyma as narrow septa. This field is traversed by one such fibrous band containing several small interlobular bile ducts (left). Infiltration by inflammatory cells is slight in this case. While the cause may be unknown, consideration should be given to the possibility of non-cirrhotic portal fibrosis with portal hypertension, especially if there be thickening of the walls of portal veins (**3.15**), a condition sometimes caused by ingestion of arsenic, copper sulphate, vinyl chloride or thorotrast. Other patients give a history of chronic active hepatitis treated with corticosteroids. If bile ductules are prominent, congenital hepatic fibrosis (**11.8**) should be considered. × 47 Hematoxylin and eosin.

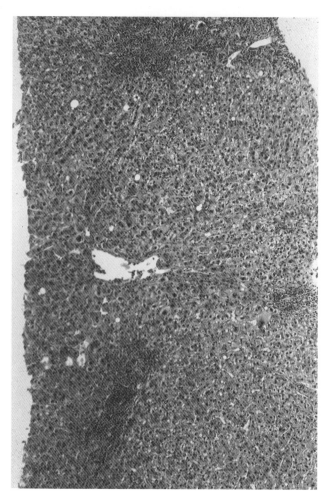

7.7 Chronic persistent hepatitis.

7.10 Chronic septal hepatitis

Fine fibrous septa bridging adjacent portal tracts or portal tracts and central veins are well shown in this reticulin-stained section. In small needle biopsies the condition can be mistaken for macronodular cirrhosis but in septal hepatitis the parenchyma usually consists of plates of single-cell thickness. × 19 Reticulin stain.

7.11 Liver in systemic lupus erythematosus

It is unusual for the liver to be seriously affected in this disease, and biopsies show only minor inflammatory changes of the non-specific reactive hepatitis pattern, as in this case with mild portal inflammation and a small focus of lobular hepatitis (arrow). Aggregates of lymphocytes are sometimes prominent. This patient did develop severe chronic active hepatitis and died of liver failure eleven years after the date of this biopsy, but such an outcome is very unusual. So-called 'lupoid' hepatitis of unknown etiology with circulating antinuclear factor and LE cells is merely a form of chronic active hepatitis already described and not the hepatic manifestation of systemic lupus erythematosus. × 50 Hematoxylin and eosin.

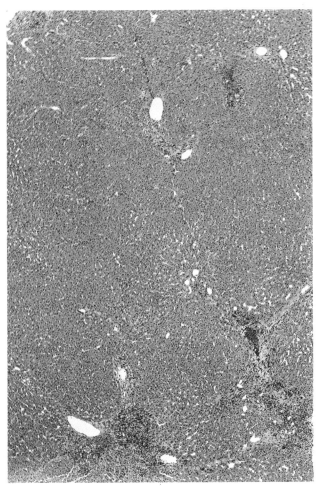

7.8 Non-specific reactive hepatitis.

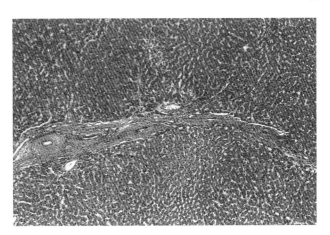

7.9 Chronic septal hepatitis.

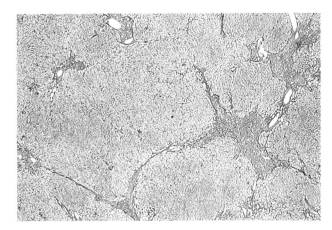

7.10 Chronic septal hepatitis.

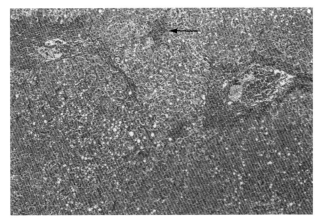

7.11 Liver in systemic lupus erythematosus.

7.12 Primary biliary cirrhosis

This liver was slightly enlarged and of firm consistency. It shows dull green discoloration due to retained bile. The surface is finely granular because of developing micronodular cirrhosis. The two depressions in the right lobe are 'cough fissures' attributed to pressure by hypertrophied diaphragmatic muscle bundles; they are an incidental finding in this case.

7.13 Primary biliary cirrhosis

This is a cut surface of the liver shown in **7.12**. Here, as in many examples of this condition, micronodular cirrhosis is less evident when compared with the appearance of the outer surface of the organ. In some cases the degree of fibrosis or cirrhosis varies from place to place, indicating the variable rate of development in different parts of the liver. In this case death occurred before the terminal fourth stage of the disease when true cirrhosis is well established. For this reason the term 'chronic non-suppurative destructive cholangitis' is more appropriate to the condition.

7.14 Primary biliary cirrhosis: stage 1 (florid bile duct lesions)

Low-power examination shows lymphocytic infiltration of portal tracts; it is often rather dense, and can amount to lymph follicle formation. Small bile ducts and ductules are absent, but there is no cholestasis. Liver parenchymal damage is also inconspicuous but in some cases there may be small foci of necrosis, minor degrees of piecemeal destruction and Kupffer cell hyperplasia. Small non-caseating granulomas are not infrequent, usually in or near widened portal tracts, and one is seen just above and to the left of centre. Since the portal changes are of irregular distribution and severity, parts of a biopsy may show little or no abnormality, especially in early cases. × 45 Hematoxylin and eosin.

7.15 Primary biliary cirrhosis: stage 1

Degeneration of bile duct epithelium is the essential lesion of the disease and is distributed in an irregular segmental fashion in interlobular and septal ducts. In this field the duct epithelial cells are swollen and irregular in shape and a few are undergoing necrosis. Other ducts may exhibit epithelial proliferation so that the lining can be several cells thick. There may also be points of rupture with destruction of basement membrane. This damaged duct is surrounded by a halo of plasma cells and these in turn by a thicker rim of lymphocytes. Neutrophils and eosinophils are sometimes present and small granulomas appear in close association. There is no conspicuous piecemeal destruction of adjacent hepatocytes. × 117 Hematoxylin and eosin.

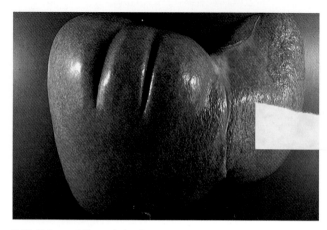

7.12 Primary biliary cirrhosis.

7.16 Primary biliary cirrhosis: stage 1

A small non-caseating granuloma is seen in close proximity to a portal tract made conspicuous by lymphocytic infiltration. Note the absence of bile ducts and ductules which in itself is suggestive of the correct diagnosis. There is no cholestasis. A few hepatocytes show hydropic and hyaline degeneration but piecemeal loss is relatively mild compared with typical chronic active hepatitis. In a minority of cases there is more severe periportal inflammation with fibrosis and loss of adjacent parenchyma, so that the distinction from chronic active hepatitis can be difficult to determine. × 75 Hematoxylin and eosin.

7.17 Primary biliary cirrhosis: stage 1

Apart from discrete granulomas there may be small aggregates of pale macrophages swollen with ingested lipid droplets (xanthoma cells). A small cluster is present in this field in close relationship to a portal tract (top left). × 300 Hematoxylin and eosin.

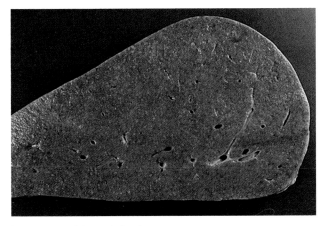

7.13 Primary biliary cirrhosis.

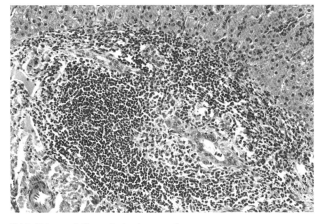

7.15 Primary biliary cirrhosis: stage 1.

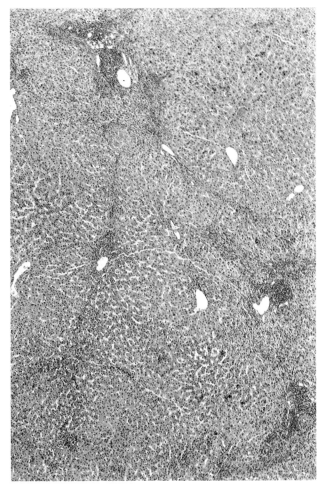

7.14 Primary biliary cirrhosis: stage 1 (florid bile duct lesions).

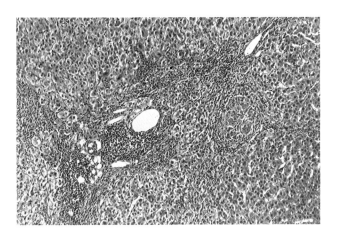

7.16 Primary biliary cirrhosis: stage 1.

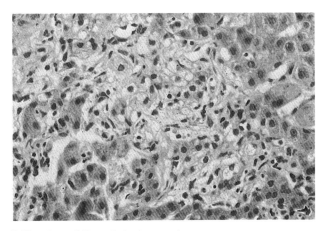

7.17 Primary biliary cirrhosis: stage 1.

7.18 Primary biliary cirrhosis: stage 2 (bile ductular proliferation)

The portal tract (below) shows the same dense lympho-cytic infiltration and absence of bile ducts as already described (**7.14**). That in the upper part of the field is widened by bile ductular proliferation, which is generally regarded as a somewhat later stage in the development of the disease. There is mild piecemeal necrosis adjacent to the upper tract and a small focus of lobular hepatocyte loss (arrow). × 88 Hematoxylin and eosin.

7.19 Primary biliary cirrhosis: stage 2

As the disease advances there is damage to hepato-cytes adjacent to the inflamed portal areas, made evident by some piecemeal necrosis together with hydropic and hyaline degeneration. Mallory bodies are present in this peripheral zone (arrows). Their distribution differs from that of Mallory bodies in alcoholic hepatitis which is more irregular throughout the liver lobules or maximal in the centrilobular zones. Cuffing of hyaline hepatocytes by neutrophil poly-morphs, which may occur in severe alcoholic cases, is not seen in primary biliary cirrhosis. × 146 Hema-toxylin and eosin.

7.20 Primary biliary cirrhosis: stage 2

Bile-capillary cholestasis is another feature of ad-vancing cases and has a peripheral distribution in the lobule, the result presumably of mechanical inter-ference with drainage of bile into portal tracts where there is fibrosis and distortion or destruction of bile channels. In this field several small dark plugs of bile pigment can be seen on either side of the chronically inflamed and fibrotic portal tract. At higher magnifi-cation it may be possible to detect small granules of pigment in peripheral hepatocytes. These can be due to either bile or copper. Note that centrilobular bile-capillary cholestasis (**2.2**) does not occur in primary biliary cirrhosis. × 88 Hematoxylin and eosin.

7.21 Primary biliary cirrhosis: stage 2

Occasionally, inspissated bile pigment is seen within proliferated bile ductules, a prominent feature of this case. These structures lie at the edge of a fibrotic portal tract in the centre of the field. Note the absence of an interlobular bile duct. Bile infarcts and bile lakes adjacent to portal tracts are other unusual manifesta-tions of primary biliary cirrhosis, being commoner in cases of large bile duct obstruction (chapter 2). × 81 Hematoxylin and eosin.

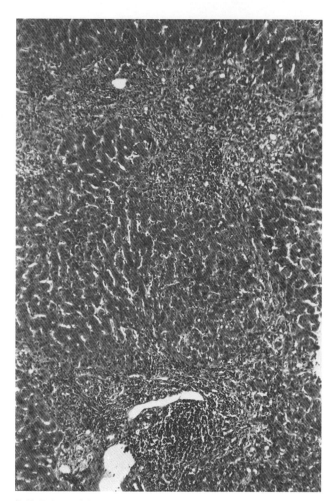

7.18 Primary biliary cirrhosis: stage 2 (bile ductular proliferation).

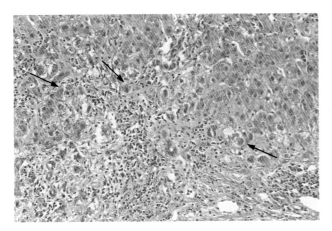

7.19 Primary biliary cirrhosis: stage 2.

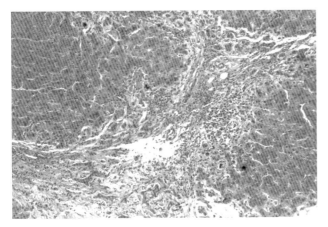

7.20 Primary biliary cirrhosis: stage 2.

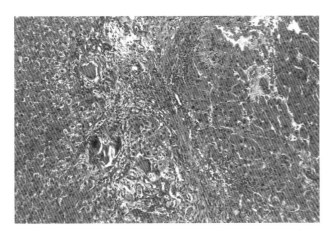

7.21 Primary biliary cirrhosis: stage 2.

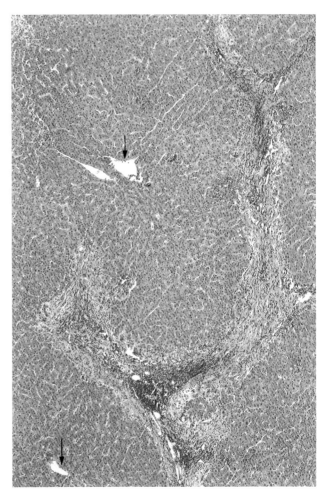

7.22 Primary biliary cirrhosis: stage 3 (portal and septal fibrosis).

7.22 Primary biliary cirrhosis: stage 3 (portal and septal fibrosis)

As the disease progresses further, fibrous septa become more conspicuous and tend to form bridges between adjacent portal tracts, leaving the central veins (arrows) unaffected. The development of a monolobular pattern of fibrosis is evident in this section. While a similar fibrotic pattern is seen in biliary disease secondary to extrahepatic obstruction, the rather dense portal lymphocytic infiltration and lack of bile ducts in this case are typical of the primary type of lesion. Proliferation of bile ductules diminishes at this stage. ×45 Hematoxylin and eosin.

7.23 Primary biliary cirrhosis: stage 4 (true cirrhosis)

In the terminal stage there is nodular regeneration of surviving parenchyma forming a rather fine mono-lobular type of cirrhosis. Some nodules may be rather irregular in shape and give a jigsaw pattern to liver parenchyma. Each nodule is delineated by a margin of hydropic hepatocytes in which bile and copper pigmentation and Mallory body formation may be seen at higher magnification. Note the persistence of prominent lymphocytic aggregates and absence of bile ducts. Granulomas are occasionally seen even at this late stage. × 36 Van Gieson's stain and hematoxylin.

7.24 Primary biliary cirrhosis: copper retention

In this post-mortem preparation stained with rubeanic acid, there is a striking deposition of copper in hepatocytes at the periphery of the cirrhotic nodules. Copper can be demonstrated frequently in hepatocytes in primary biliary cirrhosis especially in the more advanced cases although the amount here is unusually great. Its presence in relationship to hepatic fibrogenesis in primary biliary cirrhosis is still uncertain. × 47 Rubeanic acid and neutral red.

7.25 Cryptogenic cirrhosis

There is indeterminate cirrhosis with loss of normal liver architecture, the parenchyma consisting of nodules separated by red fibrous bands. There is chronic inflammation in the fibrous areas especially in the centre of the field. The clinical history of this case was suggestive of preceding idiopathic chronic active hepatitis. × 45 Van Gieson's stain and hematoxylin.

7.26 Cryptogenic cirrhosis

The liver of a patient who suffered from portal hypertension over many years and who died of liver failure. The cause of liver disease which resulted in cirrhosis was not discovered. Cryptogenic cirrhosis is often macronodular but in this case the pattern is typical of neither the macronodular nor the micronodular variety; such cases are usually described as indeterminate.

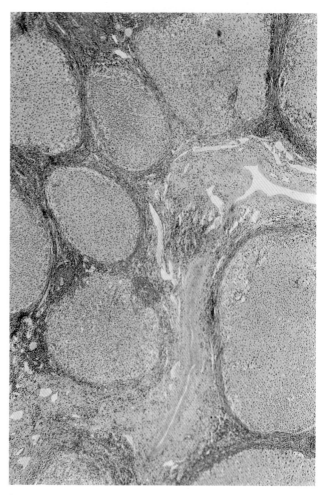

7.23 Primary biliary cirrhosis: stage 4 (true cirrhosis).

7.27 Cryptogenic cirrhosis

A macronodular pattern is well demonstrated in this section stained for reticulin. Note that the larger nodules contain diminutive portal tracts (arrow) and are traversed partly or completely by fine fibrous septa. These may represent sites of fissuring in tissue undergoing nodular expansion and are referred to as 'stress fissures'. Staining for reticulin may help also to delineate double cell liver plates which are evidence of parenchymal regeneration. × 30 Reticulin stain.

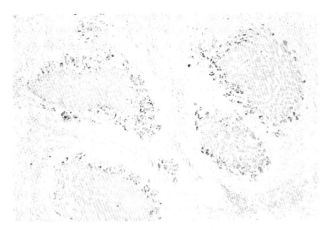

7.24 Primary biliary cirrhosis: copper retention.

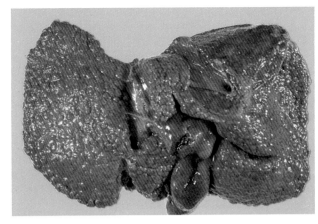

7.26 Cryptogenic cirrhosis.

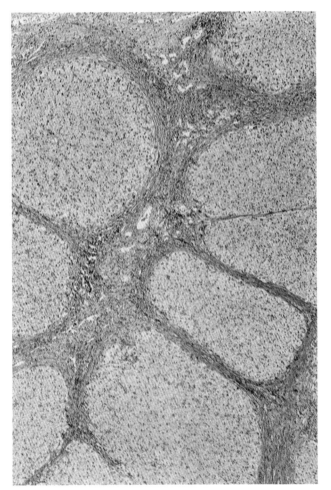

7.25 Cryptogenic cirrhosis.

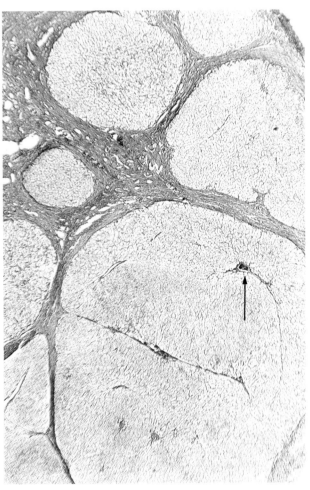

7.27 Cryptogenic cirrhosis.

7.28 Indian childhood cirrhosis

In this disease there is chronic hepatitis which leads to a micronodular type of cirrhosis. Hyaline degeneration of hepatocytes is conspicuous, a large proportion of liver cells in this field containing Mallory bodies, while some others are hydropic. Very fine connective tissue fibres separate individual hepatocytes or small groups of these cells, and this is another characteristic feature of the disease. Unlike typical alcoholic liver disease, fatty change is minimal. ×187 Hematoxylin and eosin.

7.29 Indian childhood cirrhosis

Many hepatocytes are atrophic and some especially on the left contain hyalin which stains intensely red. Fine fibres of blue staining collagen are numerous. ×234 Martius-scarlet-blue.

7.30 Types of connective tissue in chronic hepatitis

Various types of collagen and non-collagenous connective tissue components such as fibronectin and laminin may be identified in sections of fibrotic liver by means of immunohistochemistry. A reticulin stain can be helpful, as illustrated here, in distinguishing type I from type III collagen; vertical grey fibres of the former are seen on the right, while the exaggerated reticulin pattern on the left consists of black type III fibres. ×300 Reticulin stain.

7.31 Elastic fibre formation in hepatic fibrosis

The connective tissue below the parenchymatous nodule in this cirrhotic liver contains elastic fibres which have been stained a dark brown colour with orcein. This is thought to indicate active fibrogenesis. ×146 Orcein.

7.32 Elastic fibre formation in hepatic fibrosis

In this field elastic fibres stained with orcein are confined to the walls of blood vessels in the portal tract (right). The absence of similar fibres in the areas of fibrosis indicates that the latter have arisen through condensation of pre-existing stroma. This has occurred here in relation to bridging necrosis complicating viral hepatitis. Positive staining of irregularly distributed groups of hepatocytes is indicative of hepatitis B surface antigen (**6.24**). ×47 Orcein.

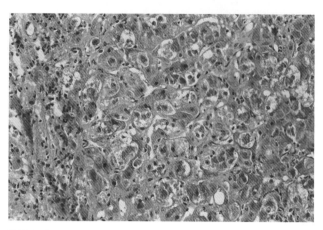

7.28 Indian childhood cirrhosis.

7.33 Sulphated mucopolysaccharide formation in chronic hepatitis

This coarse-grain autoradiograph was prepared from a fresh primary biliary cirrhosis biopsy incubated in tissue culture medium which contained radioactive (S35) sulphate for thirty minutes prior to fixation and preparation of tissue sections. The black grains represent S35 incorporated into mucopolysaccharide during this incubation period, an activity carried out almost entirely by connective tissue cells which are also synthesizing collagen. This activity is readily apparent in the expanded portal tract on the right and to a less extent along sinusoidal walls. By contrast normal fresh liver treated in this way shows no S35 uptake. Hepatic fibrogenesis as assessed by this procedure is often much greater than suspected from examination of routine histological preparations. ×47 Autoradiograph.

7.34 Fibrosis associated with bile ductular proliferation

This is part of a cirrhotic liver showing prominent bile ductular proliferation which includes small islands of epithelium and even single epithelial cells ('oval cells'). These cells are all capable of producing basement membrane with type IV collagen which will contribute to fibrogenesis in chronic liver disease. Basement membrane is demonstrated here as thin continuous purple lines which delineate these epithelial structures. ×234 Periodic acid-Schiff method and hematoxylin.

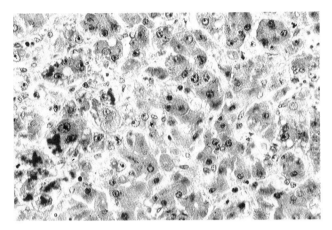

7.29 Indian childhood cirrhosis.

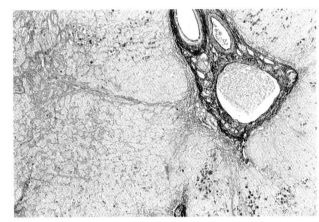

7.32 Elastic fibre formation in hepatic fibrosis.

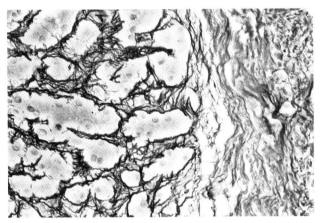

7.30 Types of connective tissue in chronic hepatitis.

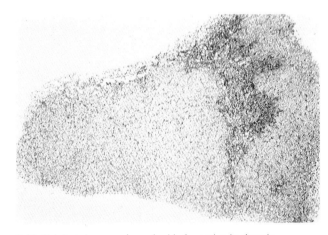

7.33 Sulphated mucopolysaccharide formation in chronic hepatitis.

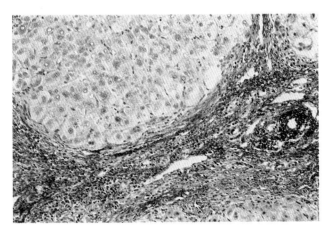

7.31 Elastic fibre formation in hepatic fibrosis.

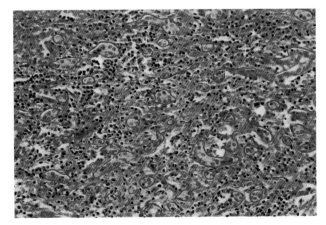

7.34 Fibrosis associated with bile ductular proliferation.

CHAPTER 8

Non-viral Infections and Infestations

8.1 Tuberculosis

Two typical granulomatous lesions are seen, consisting of epithelioid cells, multinucleated giant cells and marginal lymphocytes. The larger granuloma has a central area of caseous necrosis. These lesions are distributed in a haphazard fashion throughout the liver and may coalesce to form large tuberculomas. Alternatively, with appropriate anti-tuberculosis therapy, they may resolve leaving scars which are sometimes calcified. × 47 Hematoxylin and eosin.

8.2 Tuberculosis

There are two small chronic inflammatory lesions, that on the right being a granuloma consisting of epithelioid cells, while that on the left is a collection of lymphocytes. The patient had an opportunistic tuberculous infection related to corticosteroid administration and a systemic illness which, unlike typical miliary tuberculosis, had persisted for many months. Tuberculosis must always be considered in the investigation of granulomatous hepatitis even when the lesions, as in this case, have no Langhans-type giant cells or caseation necrosis. × 94 Hematoxylin and eosin.

8.3 Brucellosis

This biopsy had several deeply-staining collections of inflammatory cells scattered throughout the liver. Two of these microgranulomas are seen here. They consist of lymphocytes, plasma cells and macrophages, but multinucleated giant cells are uncommon. Brucella organisms are detected occasionally within macrophages. This form of granulomatous hepatitis occurs in some cases of *Br. abortus* infection. *Br. melitensis* may cause a non-specific type of reactive hepatitis with Kupffer cell activity but without distinct granulomatous lesions. × 146 Hematoxylin and eosin.

8.4 Sarcoidosis

In this disease, liver biopsy very frequently shows typical non-caseating epithelioid granulomas. Three of these lesions are present in this field. Their distribution is haphazard and may include portal tracts (top right). When only the portal tracts are involved, the possibility of primary biliary cirrhosis must be considered. Schaumann bodies may be seen in giant cells but are uncommon. × 47 Hematoxylin and eosin.

8.5 Sarcoid cirrhosis

There are broad bands of vascular connective tissue infiltrated by lymphocytes and containing a number of multinucleated giant cells. These lesions develop from confluence of numerous discrete sarcoid granulomas. In advanced cases there is extensive fibrosis and disappearance of typical granulomatous lesions. Although the liver is involved very frequently in sarcoidosis it is only a small minority of patients who develop extensive fibrosis or cirrhosis with accompanying liver dysfunction and portal hypertension. × 59 Hematoxylin and eosin.

8.6 Granulomatous hepatitis

This term should be reserved for those cases, which are not infrequent, in whom none of the numerous recognized infective or toxic causes of liver granulomas can be identified, and in whom the Kveim test for sarcoidosis is negative. In this illustration there are numerous small collections of epithelioid cells and a prominent infiltration by eosinophils, the latter being an inconstant feature of these cases. Their presence here is suggestive of an infestation such as ascariasis with destruction and disappearance of larvae, but this was never substantiated in this patient. × 117 Hematoxylin and eosin.

8.1 Tuberculosis.

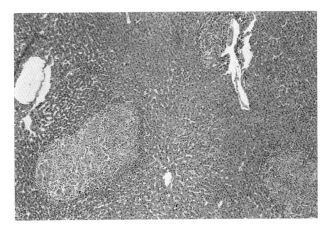

8.4 Sarcoidosis.

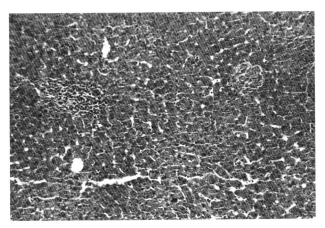

8.2 Tuberculosis.

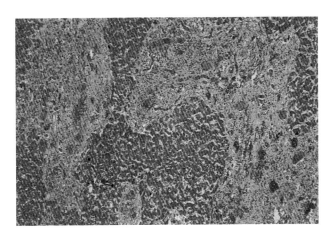

8.5 Sarcoid cirrhosis.

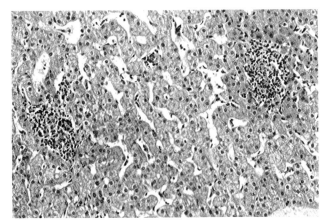

8.3 Brucellosis.

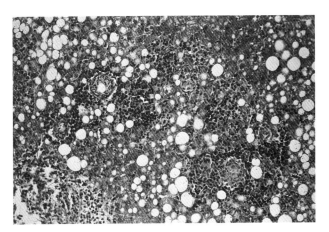

8.6 Granulomatous hepatitis.

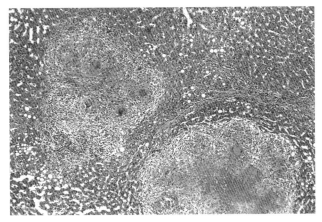

8.7 Syphilis: gumma

The lesion is a large dull-yellow nodule with a little adherent omental fat situated near the centre of the specimen. The remainder of the liver appears cirrhotic but nodular parenchymal regeneration was not evident histologically, and the septal fibrosis which was present may have been induced by arsenical therapy. It is doubtful whether true cirrhosis can ever be attributed directly to acquired syphilitic infection. Coarse scarring may ensue from fibrotic healing of gummas and a few may undergo calcification.

8.8 Syphilis: gumma

This section is from the edge of a necrotic lesion, about 5 cm in diameter, situated within the liver. The margin, which traverses the centre of the field, consists of vascular fibrous tissue in which some bile ducts are entrapped. Multinucleated giant cells and endarteritis are additional microscopic features of gumma, but are not seen in this field. × 45 Hematoxylin and eosin.

8.9 Syphilis: hepar lobatum

The liver is greatly distorted but there is no true cirrhosis as the parenchyma situated between the scars and fissures has normal microanatomical features. Scarring is regarded as a sequel to the healing of intrahepatic gummas. There is fibrous thickening of the liver capsule which was adherent to omentum, diaphragm and anterior abdominal wall.

8.10 Syphilis: congenital infection

The liver parenchyma consists of small groups of atrophic hepatocytes separated by much loose areolar connective tissue. This pericellular type of fibrosis is characteristic of the disease. In the centre of the field there is a miliary gumma with a necrotic core and margin of chronic inflammatory cells. Small gummas such as this are numerous in some cases. There is a little generalized inflammatory cell infiltration. In older children the development of a larger hepatic gumma may be the first indication of congenital syphilis. × 75 Hematoxylin and eosin.

8.11 Syphilis: congenital infection

Staining of liver sections in congenital syphilis by the Levaditi method reveals spirochaetes as short black tortuous filaments. They are present in very large numbers throughout the organ. × 338 Levaditi's method.

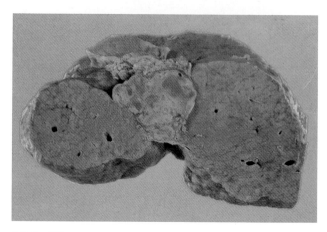

8.7 Syphilis: gumma.

8.12 Leptospirosis

An autopsy specimen showing remarkable dissociation of liver cell plates and separation of hepatocytes. Hepatocytes have prominent nuclei and nucleoli and some are binucleate. A few are clearly necrotic with fragmentation or loss of nuclei. There is no inflammatory cell infiltrate in this field but neutrophil polymorphs can be prominent in sinusoids. These changes are very characteristic of the infection but are not invariably present even in fatal cases, in some of whom liver histology may be normal. Such patients may have severe renal tubular injury while their jaundice may be due, at least in part, to hemolysis in extensive hemorrhagic lesions. × 234 Hematoxylin and eosin.

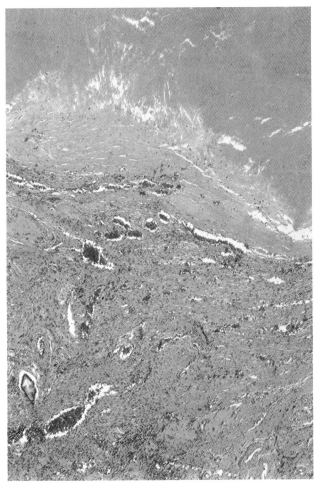

8.8 Syphilis: gumma.

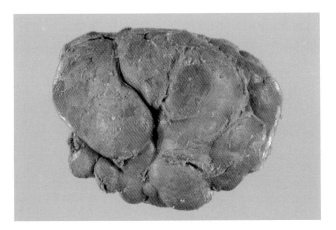

8.9 Syphilis: hepar lobatum.

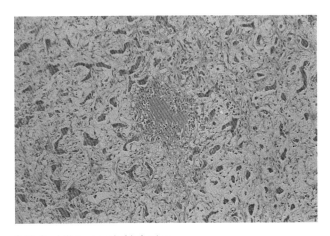

8.10 Syphilis: congenital infection.

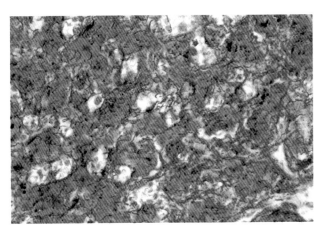

8.11 Syphilis: congenital infection.

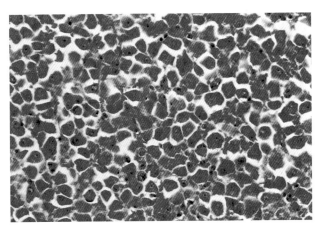

8.12 Leptospirosis.

8.13 Actinomycosis

This slice of liver shows several large honeycomb abscesses which contained purulent fluid with 'sulphur granules'.

8.14 Actinomycosis

Part of a large liver abscess found at autopsy. Degenerate hepatic tissue is on the right. On the left there are pus and three small dark colonies of Gram-positive *Actinomyces israelii*, the 'sulphur granules', which can be seen on naked-eye examination. In more chronic cases there are numerous macrophages and granulomatous tissue leading to extensive fibrosis. × 117 Gram's stain for organisms.

8.15 Actinomycosis

These are two colonies of actinomyces, each with a cuff of acute inflammatory cells. The organisms which consist of clumps of filamentous hyphae are stained by the periodic acid-Schiff technique. × 187 Periodic acid-Schiff method and hematoxylin.

8.16 Histoplasmosis

There are numerous small spherical spores of *Histoplasma capsulatum* which stain with hematoxylin. They are situated within the vacuolated cytoplasm of Kupffer cells, one of which is indicated by an arrow. Adjacent hepatocytes are atrophic, possibly from pressure of the adjacent swollen Kupffer cells. There is hardly any inflammatory response but small granulomas can occur in this infection, which commonly involves the liver. × 300 Hematoxylin and eosin.

8.17 Cryptococcosis

There is an area of necrosis in the centre and right of this field containing numerous spherical yeasts (*Cryptococcus neoformans*) but relatively little inflammatory response. Occasionally these lesions are widespread and cause serious liver damage, usually in patients with immune deficiency, but in most cases the brunt of the infection falls on the pulmonary and nervous systems. × 146 Hematoxylin and eosin.

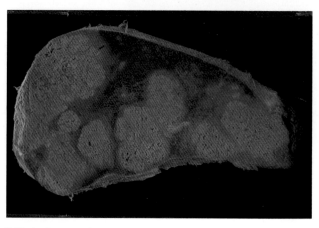

8.13 Actinomycosis.

8.18 Focal hepatic necrosis in septicemia

A fatal case of staphylococcal septicemia in which the cut surface of the congested liver shows several small dark foci of necrosis two of which are indicated by arrows. In some cases these foci may contain purulent fluid. Similar necrotic lesions may be found in streptococcal septicemia and in lobar pneumonia. Staphylococci may also cause a large solitary pyogenic abscess in the liver (**8.25**).

8.19 Typhoid fever

The liver from a fatal case showing part of a typhoid nodule. This consists of collections of inflammatory cells, mostly monocytes, which surround a small clump of *Salmonella typhi* organisms (upper centre). It is unusual to detect these bacilli in typhoid nodules. The nodules are usually periportal in distribution. Cholangiohepatitis associated with cholecystitis and gallstones is another possible hepatic manifestation of Salmonella infections. × 146 Hematoxylin and eosin.

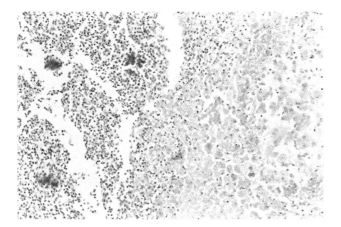

8.14 Actinomycosis.

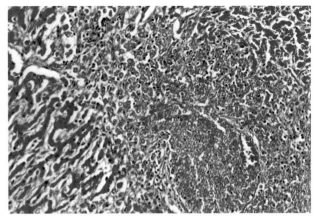

8.17 Cryptococcosis.

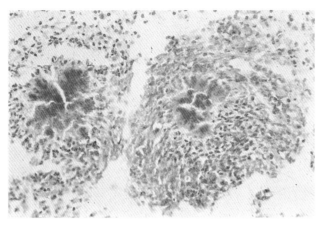

8.15 Actinomycosis.

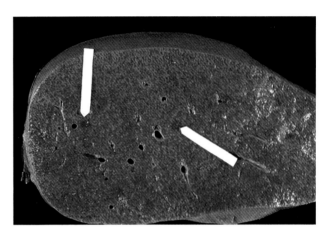

8.18 Focal hepatic necrosis in septicemia.

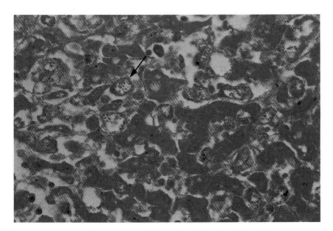

8.16 Histoplasmosis.

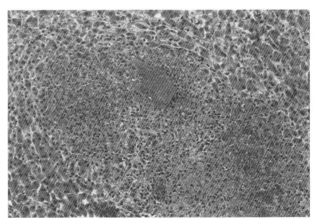

8.19 Typhoid fever.

8.20 Malaria

Lymphocytes are prominent within the hepatic sinusoids. Kupffer cells are also conspicuous because of ingested black hemozoin pigment which is a product of hemoglobin destroyed by the plasmodial organisms. It does not stain by Perls' method and is soluble in alcoholic picric acid. This pigment is found in cases of chronic malarial infection, especially in periportal Kupffer cells and in macrophages within portal tracts. It appears to be very similar to the pigment seen in the liver in bilharzial infestations, but the two differ in their ultrastructural appearances. × 220 Hematoxylin and eosin.

8.21 Liver in tropical splenomegaly ('big-spleen disease')

There is infiltration of the liver sinusoids and the portal tract (bottom right) with round cells which had the ultrastructural features of normal lymphocytes and macrophages. Malaria pigment is not present. Light-microscope appearances may suggest chronic lymphatic leukemia, but the disease occurs in malarious areas and responds to prolonged anti-malaria therapy. 'Big-spleen disease' may represent an abnormal immunological response to the infection. × 146 Hematoxylin and eosin.

8.22 Visceral Leishmaniasis (Kala-azar)

Many Leishman–Donovan bodies can be seen within swollen Kupffer cells. These bodies are round or oval and measure 2 to 4 micrometers in diameter. Each contains two small chromatin masses, but the morphology can be studied adequately only in smears of splenic or hepatic aspirates treated by a Romanovsky stain. Kupffer cell involvement is a feature of chronic cases, whereas during the acute infection, there may be hepatocyte necrosis and formation of granulomas. Extensive hepatic fibrosis may supervene. × 585 Hematoxylin and eosin.

8.23 Amebiasis

There is an area of coagulation necrosis above and to the right, and of compressed fatty liver below. There are a few lymphocytes in the marginal zone, but in the absence of secondary pyogenic infection there is often little inflammatory reaction including granulation tissue formation and subsequent fibrosis. A few amebae can just be detected as spherical and rather basophilic bodies, but they are not conspicuous at this magnification. × 117 Hematoxylin and eosin.

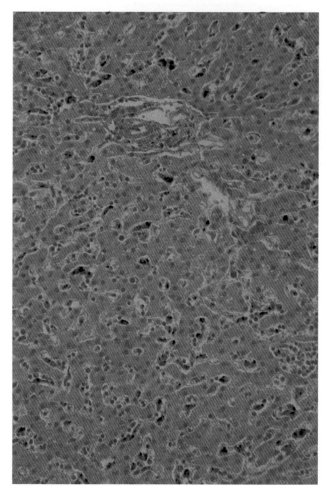

8.20 Malaria.

8.24 Amebiasis

Two pathogenic amebae (*Entameba histolytica*) are present in this field. They are detected readily because of their relatively large size and basophilic staining. They may contain ingested erythrocytes and be surrounded by a clear halo but these features are not apparent in this illustration. × 750 Hematoxylin and eosin.

8.25 Pyogenic abscess of liver

The liver contains an extensive area of suppuration and necrosis (approx. 12 × 8 cm) due to staphylococcal infection. This type of lesion may be difficult to distinguish from amebic abscess without histological and microbiological investigations. Moreover, pyogenic infection may supervene in amebic abscess following attempts at aspiration or drainage and in such cases the definition of pathogenic amebae can be difficult.

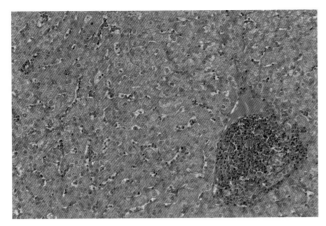

8.21 Liver in tropical splenomegaly ('big-spleen disease').

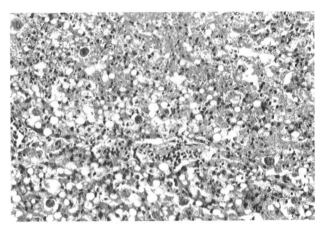

8.23 Amebiasis.

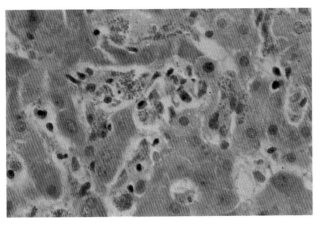

8.22 Visceral Leishmaniasis (Kala-azar).

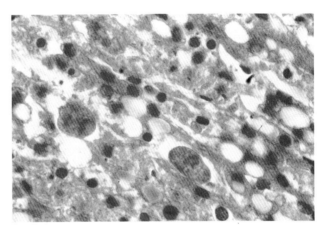

8.24 Amebiasis.

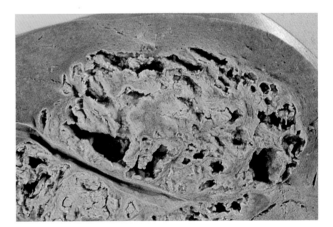

8.25 Pyogenic abscess of liver.

8.26 Subphrenic abscess

The space between the elevated diaphragm and upper surface of the liver contained purulent material. The underlying liver parenchyma is pale with focal congestion, and histological examination of this part revealed acute inflammation and some hemorrhagic necrosis. From a case of chronic peptic ulcer with a leaking perforation.

8.27 Schistosomiasis (Bilharziasis)

This liver biopsy from a case of chronic *Schistosoma mansoni* infestation shows a distorted schistosoma egg which has provoked a granulomatous reaction. The granuloma contains macrophages, which may be multinucleated, and there is an outer concentric rim of fibroblasts and collagen fibres, but very few lymphocytes. These ova are derived via the portal blood from adult worms which inhabit the mesenteric vessels of the patient. When viable the eggs provoke an inflammatory response which includes infiltration by numerous eosinophils. After death, as in this case, they become distorted with loss of the characteristic lateral spine on the outer surface, and a foreign-body type of granulomatous reaction develops. Eventually these lesions are completely fibrous or calcified. When there is heavy infestation, the fibrous response to the ova can be extensive and lead to extensive scarring along portal tracts ('pipestem fibrosis'). × 146 Hematoxylin and eosin.

8.28 Hydatid disease

There is a large intrahepatic cyst with a thick wall, the outer part of which consists of fibrous tissue formed by the host. The cavity contains several bulbous structures which are brood capsules from which tapeworm heads (*Echinococcus granulosus*) were recovered.

This was an incidental finding in an elderly man dying of an unrelated pulmonary infection. These cysts can reach a large size and rupture into the peritoneal cavity, causing a severe allergic response and dissemination of the disease throughout the abdomen. Secondary infection with pyogenic bacteria may also occur, probably via the biliary tract. Hydatid liver develops by ingestion of food contaminated with dog feces as the small adult tapeworms inhabit dog intestine. In turn the dogs obtain the larvae by eating raw offal of various animals which contain these cysts.

8.29 Clonorchiasis

This shows a transverse section through two flat trematode worms—flukes (*Clonorchis sinensis*)—lying within a dilated septal bile duct. Intestinal canals lined by simple columnar epithelium and vitelline glands are seen in both worms. Note the adenomatous hyperplasia of the host bile duct mucosa. This change may be related to the development of cholangiocarcinoma in some of these cases. This infestation occurs in the Orient where pyogenic cholangitis is also common. Both conditions may co-exist or occur separately. Infestation is derived from fish consumed raw or insufficiently cooked. × 35 Hematoxylin and eosin.

8.30 Toxocariasis

Fragments of degenerate larvae of *Toxocara canis* have induced a granulomatous response with multinucleated giant cells, macrophages and lymphocytes. Some fibrinoid material is also present. Toxocariasis is a rare disease occurring in children who become infested by ingestion of the nematode ova which are excreted in the feces of dogs or cats. The adult worms inhabit the intestines of these animals. × 146 Hematoxylin and eosin.

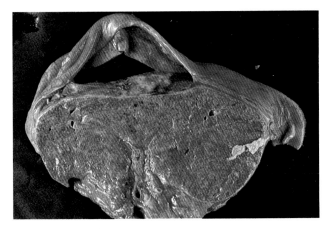

8.26 Subphrenic abscess.

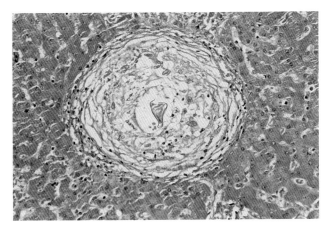

8.27 Schistosomiasis (Bilharziasis).

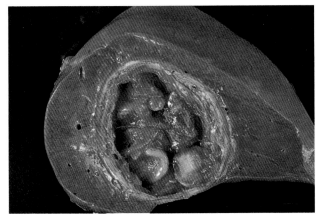

8.28 Hydatid disease.

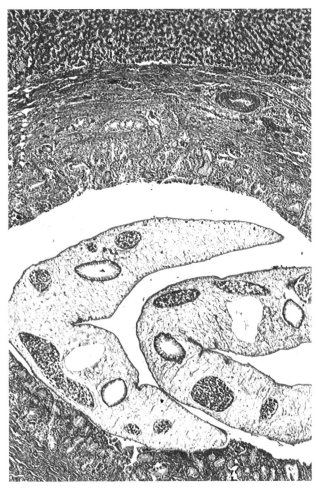

8.29 Clonorchiasis.

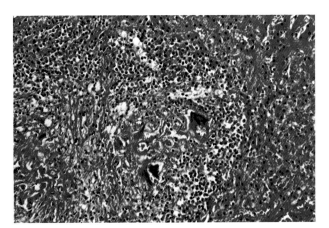

8.30 Toxocariasis.

CHAPTER 9

Metabolic Disorders

9.1 Primary hemochromatosis

There is brown discoloration of the liver due to large amounts of hemosiderin pigment. There is also micronodular cirrhosis which gives the surface a fine granular appearance. Established cirrhosis of this type is a late manifestation of the disease.

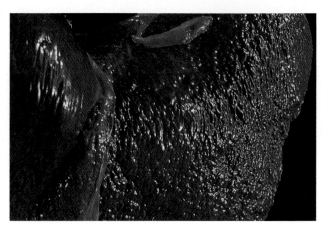

9.1 Primary hemochromatosis.

9.2 Primary hemochromatosis

Portions of liver and pancreas give an intensely positive Prussian blue reaction for hemosiderin. There is similar involvement of the parenchyma of many other organs, such as endocrine glands, gastric mucosa, sweat glands and heart. The liver contains several nodules of primary carcinoma which are unstained. The incidence of this tumour is relatively high in hemochromatosis (**10.30**).

9.3 Primary hemochromatosis

Hemosiderin within hepatocytes is not seen readily at this low magnification, but is conspicuous in portal tract macrophages. There is portal and septal fibrosis which, at this relatively early stage of the disease, has a characteristic 'holly leaf' pattern. × 45 Hematoxylin and eosin.

9.4 Primary hemochromatosis: developing cirrhosis

All hepatocytes give a positive Prussian blue reaction for hemosiderin. The parenchyma has a nodular appearance where it abuts on broad bands of fibrous tissue. At the later stage of true cirrhosis the parenchyma consists entirely of small discrete nodules. The cirrhosis is usually of micronodular pattern but can be macronodular. × 47 Perls' method and neutral red.

9.5 Primary hemochromatosis: cirrhosis

At this magnification small granules of hemosiderin are seen in hepatocytes and the epithelium of some bile ductules situated within a broad band of fibrous tissue. In some cases iron-containing pigment is encrusted on the collagen fibres of the fibrous septa. × 117 Perls' method and neutral red.

9.6 Primary hemochromatosis

The distribution of hemosiderin in Kupffer cells is irregular in primary hemochromatosis. In this field the Kupffer cells (arrows) have no pigment although the hepatocytes are heavily laden. × 300 Perls' method and neutral red.

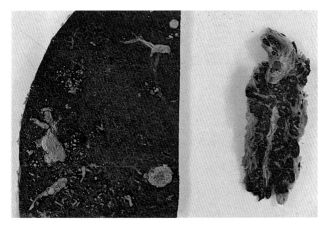

9.2 Primary hemochromatosis.

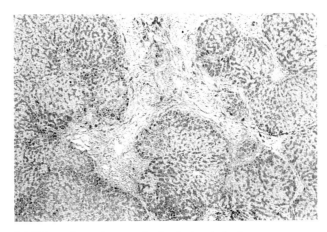

9.4 Primary hemochromatosis: developing cirrhosis.

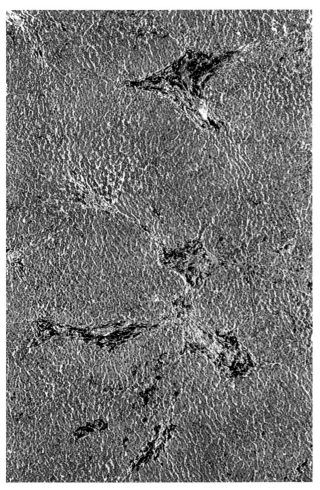

9.3 Primary hemochromatosis.

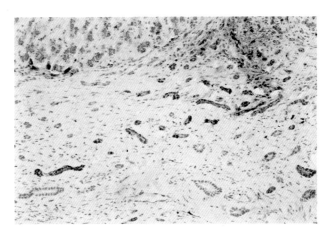

9.5 Primary hemochromatosis: cirrhosis.

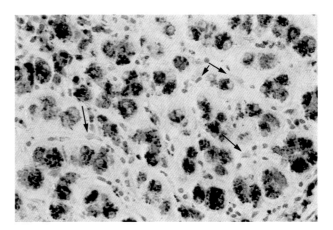

9.6 Primary hemochromatosis.

9.7 Secondary hemochromatosis

The liver from a patient with refractory anemia who had received numerous blood transfusions over many years. Hemosiderin is present in hepatocytes but is not seen readily at this low magnification. It is prominent is Kupffer cells and portal tract macrophages (compare 9.6). There is diffuse fibrosis which could proceed to a micronodular type of cirrhosis. The fibrosis appears active with inflammatory cells in the stroma and some destruction of adjacent hepatocytes (fibrosis or cirrhosis is usually relatively inactive in primary hemochromatosis). ×71 Hematoxylin and eosin.

9.8 Secondary hemochromatosis

Part of the specimen shown in 9.7 at higher magnification. In the centre of the field is a wide fibrous septum with numerous fibroblasts and some lymphocytes. Hemosiderin pigment is prominent within macrophages but is not encrusted on collagen fibres as in some cases of primary hemochromatosis. ×146 Hematoxylin and eosin.

9.9 Hemosiderin in hepatitis

In certain types of hepatitis such as those due to alcohol and porphyria, hemosiderin may be demonstrated in liver cells. In this case of alcoholic cirrhosis, hemosiderin is most prominent at the periphery of nodules, and this helps in distinguishing the condition from primary hemochromatosis in which the distribution is more diffuse (9.4). Iron pigment is not encrusted on fibrous septa in such cases, but this need not be seen in primary hemochromatosis. ×45 Perls' method and neutral red.

9.10 Liver parenchymal hemosiderosis

Hemosiderin is present in hepatocytes and is most intense at the periphery of the lobule (above). There is no fibrosis. Compare the hemosiderin giving a positive Prussian blue reaction with the brown granules of lipofuscin in centrilobular hepatocytes (below). The cause of excessive iron deposition in the liver of this patient was not known. Possibly some of these cases are in an early stage of hemochromatosis with abnormal absorption of iron from the bowel. Some others suffer from anemia with disordered erythropoiesis, such as pernicious anemia. ×177 Perls' method and neutral red.

9.11 Kupffer cell hemosiderosis

The Kupffer cells give a positive Prussian blue reaction. In contrast to primary hemochromatosis they are involved uniformly throughout the liver, while the hepatocytes contain no hemosiderin. There are many

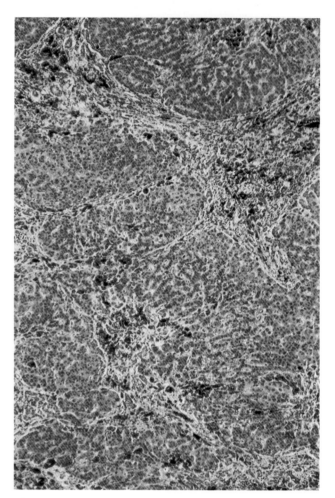

9.7 Secondary hemochromatosis.

causes for this condition including severe hemolytic anemia, blood transfusion, parenteral injection of iron compounds and extramedullary hematopoiesis. Hemosiderin may be found in association with ceroid pigment in Kupffer cells during recovery from various types of hepatocyte injury such as viral hepatitis (6.15). Its presence in anemia associated with chronic inflammatory and neoplastic diseases seems to indicate a failure of iron release and reutilization in these cases. ×187 Perls' method and neutral red.

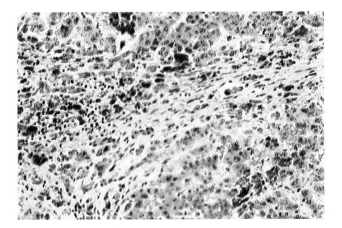

9.8 Secondary hemochromatosis.

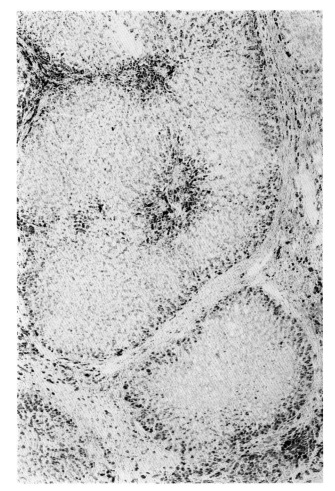

9.9 Hemosiderin in hepatitis.

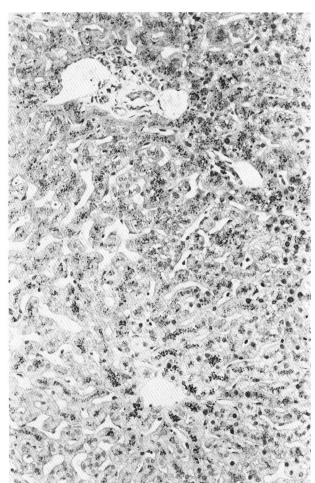

9.10 Liver parenchymal hemosiderosis.

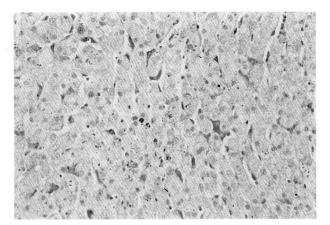

9.11 Kupffer cell hemosiderosis.

9.12 Wilson's disease

An advanced case with macronodular cirrhosis which, in the absence of copper demonstrable by special staining methods, has no features specific for Wilson's disease. Septal inflammation persists but bile ductular proliferation is not conspicuous. Cirrhosis is preceded by focal necrosis, fatty change which may be severe, and portal and periportal inflammation with cholangiolar proliferation. Therefore the resemblance to alcoholic hepatitis can be close. In some cases with piecemeal necrosis the appearances are indistinguishable from chronic active hepatitis, and Wilson's disease must be considered in the investigation of chronic hepatitis, especially in young patients. Kupffer cells may be prominent and contain hemosiderin, probably the result of incidents of hemolysis. ×30 Hematoxylin and eosin.

9.13 Wilson's disease

In both the precirrhotic and the cirrhotic stages, vacuolation of hepatocyte nuclei and hyaline degeneration of cytoplasm may be seen. The former is evident in this field (arrows). Mallory bodies when present strengthen the resemblance to alcoholic liver disease. In cirrhotic cases they are found mostly in hepatocytes at the periphery of nodules. ×187 Hematoxylin and eosin.

9.14 Wilson's disease

This section of post-mortem liver has been stained with rhodanine to show numerous red granules of copper within hepatocytes. The demonstration of copper in the liver by histochemical methods is very variable in Wilson's disease, and a negative result does not exclude this diagnosis, which can be made from the results of quantitative studies of the element in biopsy material and by the demonstration of low levels of serum ceruloplasmin. In cirrhotic cases the amount of copper demonstrated histochemically may vary greatly between different nodules. ×146 Rhodanine and hematoxylin.

9.15 Calcinosis of liver

Metastatic deposits of calcium may be seen in the liver of patients with severe hypercalcemia. The calcium salts form dark granules in the centres of liver lobules where the hepatocytes are either atrophic or have disappeared. ×71 Hematoxylin and eosin.

9.16 Calcinosis of liver

The same specimen as illustrated in **9.15** treated by von Kossa's method. Calcium salts are shown as intensely black granules. ×30 von Kossa's method and neutral red.

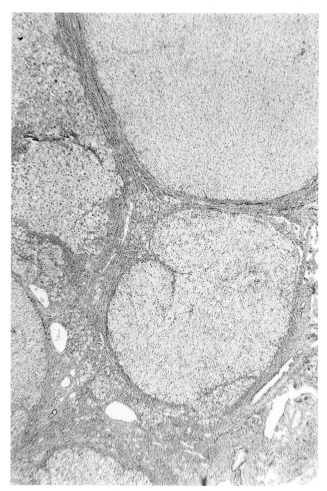

9.12 Wilson's disease.

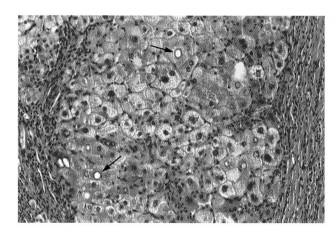

9.13 Wilson's disease.

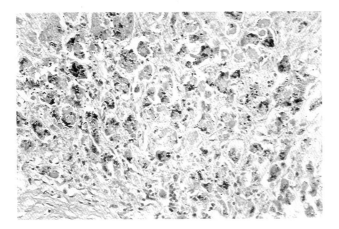

9.14 Wilson's disease.

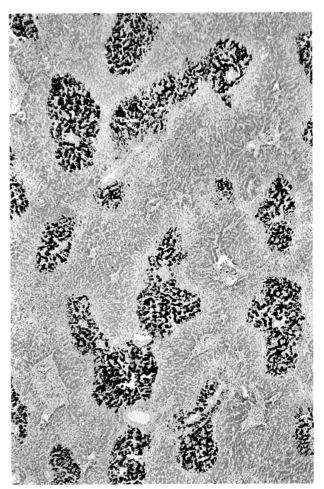

9.16 Calcinosis of liver.

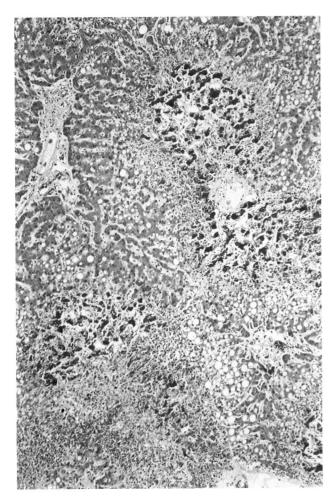

9.15 Calcinosis of liver.

9.17 Diabetes mellitus

The nuclei of some hepatocytes are vacuolated. This abnormality is seen frequently in diabetes, but may be found in other conditions such as Wilson's disease and methotrexate-induced injury. Hyaline degeneration of the hepatic arteriole (arrow) is another characteristic feature of the disease. Fatty change is slight in this case but is often present in diabetes, especially in maturity onset cases or during episodes of ketoacidosis. × 117 Hematoxylin and eosin.

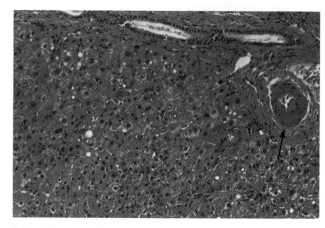

9.17 Diabetes mellitus.

9.18 Diabetes mellitus

Nuclear vacuolation is due to glycogen which is rather labile but which can be stained by the PAS method in frozen sections. This is illustrated here (arrows). Fatty change is fairly severe. Excessive quantities of glycogen may be present in hepatocytic cytoplasm in addition to nuclei. Together with retained lipid it is responsible for hepatomegaly in diabetes. × 234 Periodic acid-Schiff method and hematoxylin.

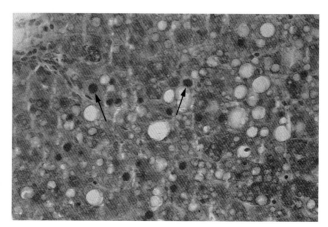

9.18 Diabetes mellitus.

9.19 Type 3 glycogen storage disease

The liver was greatly enlarged from the presence of excessive amounts of glycogen within hepatocytes. In routine paraffin sections these swollen cells with clear cytoplasm are seen to cause sinusoidal compression and present a mosaic pattern. There is a little portal fibrosis, the presence of which distinguishes type 3 from type 1 glycogen storage disease. Excess glycogen is present in the liver in other forms of glycogenosis except type 2. In type 4 it produces discrete cytoplasmic bodies which resemble Lafora bodies (**4.41**). × 75 Hematoxylin and eosin.

9.20 Galactosemia

A fairly advanced case in an infant aged five months which has progressed to cirrhosis. Nodules of surviving liver parenchyma contain purple-staining glycogen and are separated by broad bands of fibrous tissue. There is a pseudoglandular arrangement of many hepatocytes. This appearance is preceded by fatty change and proliferation of bile ducts adjacent to portal tracts. × 71 Periodic acid-Schiff method and hematoxylin.

9.21 Galactosemia

A higher magnification showing in more detail the characteristic pseudoglandular hepatocyte pattern. A few of these acinar structures contain bile pigment (arrows). There is also some proliferation of bile ductules on the left. Similar changes are found in the liver in hereditary fructose intolerance and in tyrosinemia. × 117 Hematoxylin and eosin.

9.22 Mucoviscidosis

Numerous bile ducts and ductules are distended with amorphous mucinous material of variable density and lined by flattened epithelium. These lesions are rather irregular in distribution throughout the liver and lead to a focal type of biliary cirrhosis. × 117 Hematoxylin and eosin.

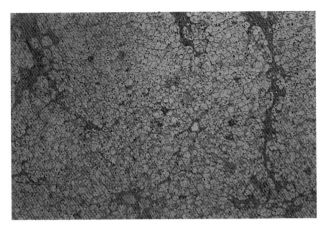

9.19 Type 3 glycogen storage disease.

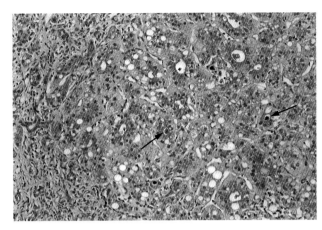

9.21 Galactosemia.

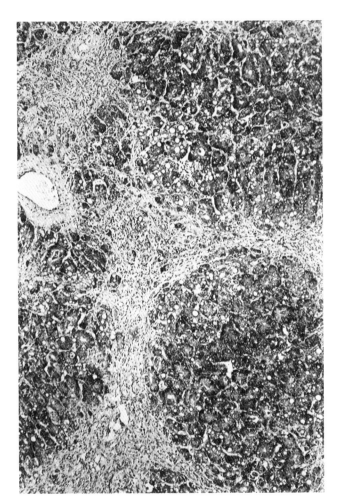

9.20 Galactosemia.

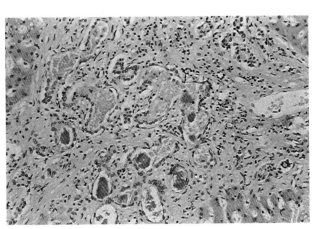

9.22 Mucoviscidosis.

9.23 Dubin–Johnson syndrome

A centrilobular zone in which hepatocytes contain prominent granules of brown pigment similar to but coarser than lipochrome granules. Although these patients have conjugated hyperbilirubinemia there is no intrahepatic cholestasis or other structural abnormality. The granules impart a dull red or grey colour to the liver which can be detected on naked-eye examination. The pigment is related to melanin and can be demonstrated by Fontana staining. Patients with Rotor syndrome have similar clinical features without hepatic pigmentation. Likewise, Gilbert's syndrome is not associated with any structural abnormality of liver detectable by light microscopy, but hyperbilirubinemia is of the unconjugated type. × 300 Hematoxylin and eosin.

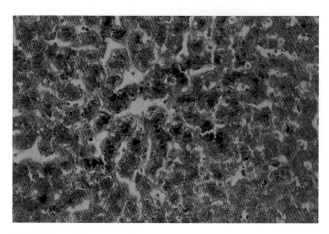

9.23 Dubin–Johnson syndrome.

9.24 Benign familial cholestatic jaundice

Bile-capillary cholestasis is seen in the centrilobular zone (right). This cannot be distinguished morphologically from the many other causes of centrilobular cholestasis (chapter 2), and the correct diagnosis is suggested by the characteristic family history of repeated attacks of cholestatic jaundice occurring throughout life and in near relatives. During these attacks liver biopsy may also show evidence of portal inflammation. Unlike Dubin–Johnson and Rotor syndromes in which some degree of hyperbilirubinemia is always present, cases of benign familial cholestatic disease have normal liver function between the episodes of jaundice. × 117 Hematoxylin and eosin.

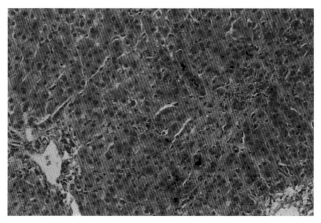

9.24 Benign familial cholestatic jaundice.

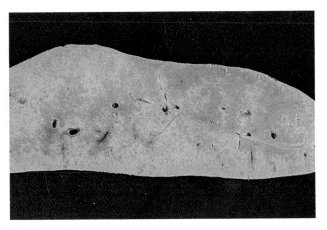

9.25 Amyloid disease.

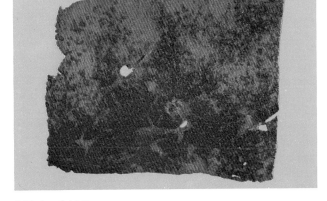

9.26 Amyloid disease.

9.25 Amyloid disease

The liver is commonly involved in both primary and secondary amyloidosis, but less frequently in the type associated with myelomatosis. This section of liver was of firm consistency and shows an irregular distribution of dull waxy material indicative of amyloid degeneration. Note the variable distribution of the disease, but distribution gives no indication of etiology.

9.26 Amyloid disease

A portion of the liver shown in **9.25** which had been immersed in Lugol's iodine solution for 5 minutes. Amyloid is stained a dark brown colour. This simple test can be carried out readily during an autopsy. Lugol's iodine.

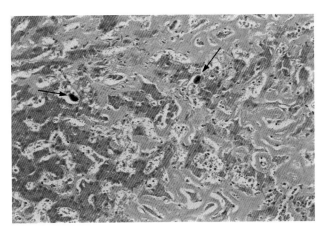

9.27 Amyloid disease.

9.27 Amyloid disease

Pale pink amyloid material is present in perisinusoidal spaces. The atrophy and loss of hepatocytes which it causes are seen especially on the right. There is rarely much evidence of liver dysfunction in these cases despite extensive parenchymal loss. Intrahepatic cholestasis is a feature of some of these cases and is present here (arrows). Fibrosis does not occur. × 117 Hematoxylin and eosin.

9.28 Amyloid disease

In this case the red-stained amyloid is confined to the walls of hepatic blood vessels. Vascular involvement alone is more common in primary amyloidosis. × 136 Sirius red and hematoxylin.

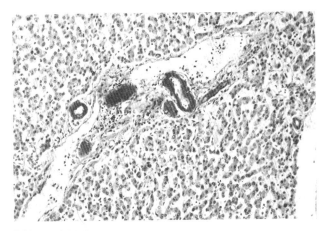

9.28 Amyloid disease.

9.29 α1-antitrypsin deficiency

A number of well-defined spherical eosinophilic bodies are seen. These represent α1-antitrypsin which is produced in the liver and which normally inhibits the action of trypsin in the blood. In this disease it is retained in excessive amount within the liver. These bodies are of variable size measuring up to 40 micrometers in diameter. There are also variable numbers within individual hepatocytes but tend to be most profuse in periportal cells. The edge of a small portal trace is seen (lower right). A number of these cases have hepatitis leading to cirrhosis, but there is no evidence of this here. × 187 Hematoxylin and eosin.

9.30 α1-antitrypsin deficiency

A severe case with cirrhosis in which many hepatocytes, especially those at the periphery of nodules contain numerous α1-antitrypsin inclusion bodies. These are PAS-positive and diastase-resistant. Fatty change is present also. The cirrhosis which develops is macronodular in type, and is sometimes characterized by very thick hyalinized collagen bands in the fibrous septa. The liver disease may be associated with abnormalities elsewhere in the body, especially pulmonary emphysema and chronic pancreatitis. An association of chronic pulmonary and hepatic disease should always raise suspicion of this diagnosis. Hepatocellular carcinoma may complicate the cirrhosis (**10.27**). × 118 Periodic acid-Schiff method and hematoxylin.

9.31 α1-antitrypsin deficiency

The diagnosis may be confirmed by immunohistochemistry, using an antibody to the retained protein in the immunoperoxidase technique. This is from the case illustrated in **9.30** and shows a positive reaction by the brown staining of the inclusion bodies. × 117 Immunoperoxidase.

9.32 Cystinosis

The liver from a case of infantile cystinosis (de Toni–Fanconi–Lignac syndrome) who died of renal failure. The alcohol-fixed tissue contains coarse grey granules of cystine within groups of enlarged Kupffer cells. The presence of cystine in the liver does not incite any inflammatory or fibrotic reaction. Cystine crystals are present in other tissues, particularly conjunctiva and cornea. There are developmental defects in renal tubules which cause serious deficiency in reabsorption of water, electrolytes and amino acids, leading to fatal renal insufficiency. Minor degrees of the disease exist, usually without hepatic involvement. × 300 Hematoxylin and eosin.

9.33 Cystinosis

Reduction of incident light by partial closure of the iris diaphragm of the microscope substage condenser brings the crystals into prominence as they refract light away from the objective. In this way it is shown that affected Kupffer cells tend to aggregate in the centre of liver lobules (above), but that there are also cystine-containing macrophages in portal tracts (below). Examination by polarized light will demonstrate the birefringent property of the crystals. Being soluble in water they may not be seen in material which has not been fixed in alcohol. × 113 Hematoxylin and eosin.

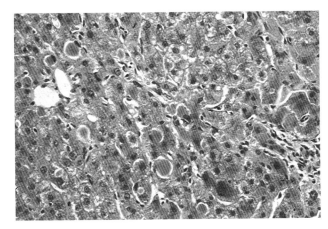

9.29 α1-antitrypsin deficiency.

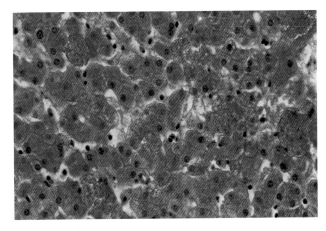

9.32 Cystinosis.

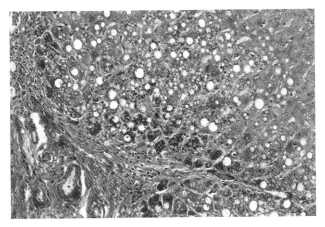

9.30 α1-antitrypsin deficiency.

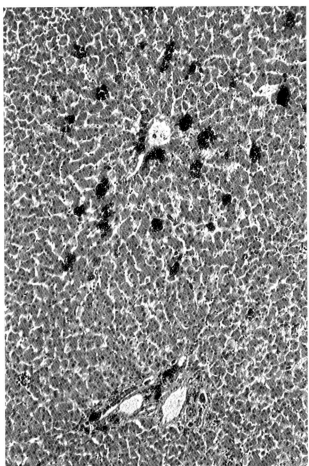

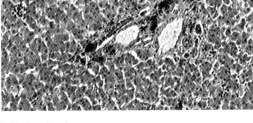

9.31 α1-antitrypsin deficiency.

9.33 Cystinosis.

9.34 Gaucher's disease

There are many Gaucher cells (upper right). These are macrophages swollen by ingested glucocerebroside; they have small round nuclei and eosinophilic cytoplasm which is either dense or vacuolated. Hepatocytes are hydropic. The distribution of these collections of Gaucher cells is haphazard in the liver lobules. By their swelling they may cause atrophy of adjacent hepatocytes and blockage of sinusoids which in some cases may lead to portal hypertension. Fibrosis and even cirrhosis have been reported occasionally but are not present in this case although the patient was adult and had suffered from the condition for many years. Gaucher cells are present in many other organs, particularly the spleen. × 117 Hematoxylin and eosin.

9.35 Gaucher's disease

The Gaucher cells give positive staining with PAS which is diastase-resistant. Small amounts of hemosiderin may also be demonstrable. × 117 Periodic acid-Schiff method and hematoxylin.

9.36 Niemann–Pick disease

There are small groups of swollen macrophages containing ingested cerebroside (sphingomyelin) which gives their cytoplasm a pale foamy appearance. In advanced cases the hepatocytes may also be involved. As in Gaucher's disease the swollen macrophage may cause hepatocyte atrophy and sinusoidal compression but these features are inconspicuous in this specimen. Again there is little tendency to the development of hepatic fibrosis and cirrhosis. There is similar involvement of other organs and splenomegaly. × 187 Hematoxylin and eosin.

9.37 Niemann–Pick disease

Unlike those in Gaucher's disease, the abnormal macrophages are PAS-negative and are highlighted in this photograph by the presence of purple-staining glycogen in hepatocytes. On the other hand they may contain ceroid pigment and give positive staining for lipid and cholesterol. × 90 Periodic acid-Schiff method and hematoxylin.

9.38 Wolman's disease

In this disease of infants the liver is grossly enlarged and pale because it contains excessive amounts of triglycerol and cholesterol, apparently the result of acid lipase deficiency. Both hepatocytes and Kupffer cells are swollen due to their high lipid content and are difficult to distinguish from each other. Note the cleft-like spaces where cholesterol has been deposited (arrows). Bile ductular proliferation and fibrosis, which are not present in this case, may occur. Cells with a similar foamy appearance are found at other sites such as bone marrow. Circulating lymphocytes have a vacuolated appearance and there is adrenal calcification. In cholesterol ester storage disease the liver biopsy appearances are similar but less severe, as are changes in other organs. × 187 Hematoxylin and eosin.

9.39 Wolman's disease

A frozen section of the same specimen illustrated in **9.38**, seen by polarized light. This demonstrates the birefringent cholesterol crystals in the liver. Dark-ground illumination.

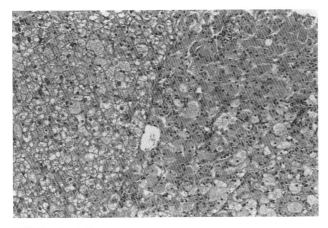

9.34 Gaucher's disease.

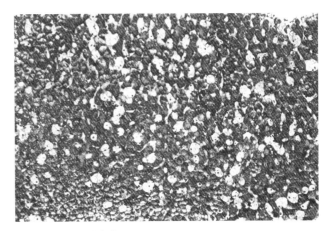

9.37 Niemann–Pick disease.

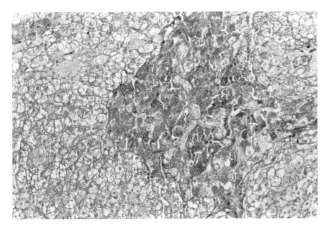

9.35 Gaucher's disease.

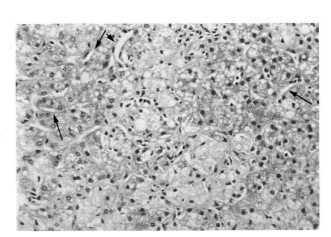

9.38 Wolman's disease.

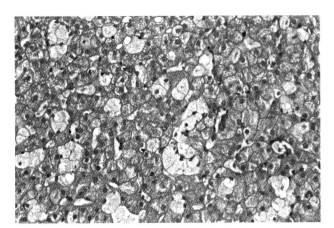

9.36 Niemann–Pick disease.

9.39 Wolman's disease.

9.40 Lipodystrophy

This biopsy shows fatty change, fibrosis and persistent hepatitis resembling alcoholic liver disease, but was from a non-alcoholic adult with severe lipodystrophy. ×87 Hematoxylin and eosin.

9.41 Lipodystrophy

A second biopsy taken from the case illustrated in **9.40** after an interval of twelve years. There is now a well-established micronodular cirrhosis. Liver disease in lipodystrophy is one of several conditions which mimic that due to alcohol (chapter 5). ×36 Martius-scarlet-blue.

9.42 Porphyria cutanea tarda

This shows red fluorescence in an unfixed dried section of liver examined by ultraviolet light in a fluorescence microscope. The reaction is most intense in cell nuclei. A similar result is obtained with unfixed tissue smears and even whole needle biopsy specimens, and is characteristic of porphyria cutanea tarda. Fluorescence is due to uroporphyrin in liver cells. Being water soluble it is not demonstrable in tissues which have been immersed in water-containing fixatives. Routine histological examination usually reveals chronic hepatitis with fatty change and siderosis which may be due, at least in part, to associated chronic alcoholism. ×188

9.43 Reye's syndrome

There is severe steatosis with large fat droplets in periportal hepatocytes and small fat droplets in centrilobular cells (centrilobular vein above and left of centre). This baby also had severe fatty change in renal tubular epithelium and died of encephalopathy. The etiology is unknown but the condition is included here as certain cases have urea cycle enzyme deficiencies e.g. reduced activity of carbamyl phosphate synthetase and ornithine transcarbamylase which cause hyperammonemia. Some cases are initiated by a virus infection especially varicella or influenza B. Some may be related to ingestion of aspirin. ×71 Hematoxylin and eosin.

9.44 Reye's syndrome

A higher magnification of the liver shown in **9.43** to illustrate large- and small-droplet fatty change affecting hepatocytes. There is no cholestasis and no hepatitis or necrosis although minor degrees of this have been noted in fatal cases. Appropriate staining usually shows glycogen depletion which correlates with hypoglycemia. ×187 Hematoxylin and eosin.

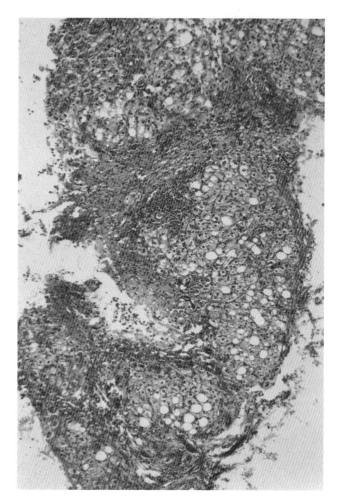

9.40 Lipodystrophy.

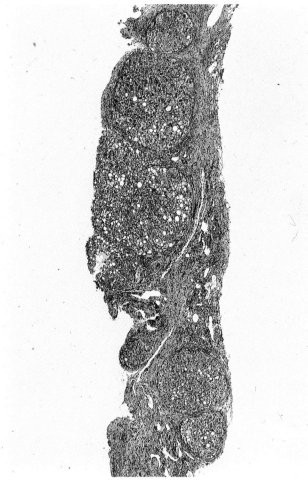

9.41 Lipodystrophy.

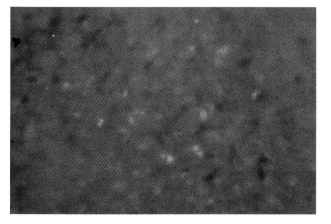

9.42 Porphyria cutanea tarda.

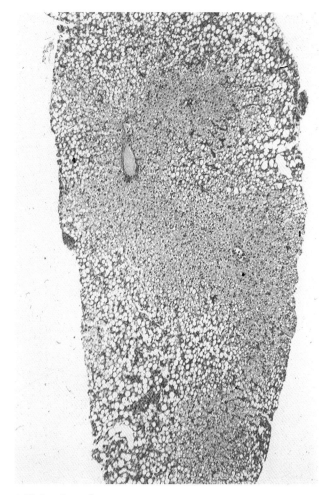

9.43 Reye's syndrome.

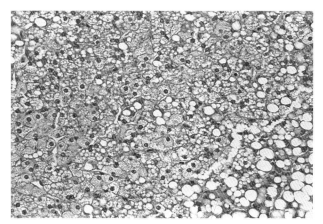

9.44 Reye's syndrome.

CHAPTER 10

Tumours

10.1 Liver cell adenoma

Part of the tumour is seen, separated from normal liver (below) by a fibrous capsule. The tumour cells resemble normal hepatocytes closely and tend to be arranged in the same trabecular fashion between thin sinusoidal channels. × 71 Hematoxylin and eosin.

10.2 Liver cell adenoma

There are small foci of hemorrhage (bottom right). These are not uncommon, especially in tumours related to intake of anabolic and contraceptive steroids. Hemorrhage can be extensive and cause serious intraperitoneal blood loss. Small blood vessels may be seen within liver cell adenomas but there are no bile ducts or portal tracts. × 30 Hematoxylin and eosin.

10.3 Focal nodular hyperplasia

This hamartomatous lesion of the liver may be mistaken for a liver cell adenoma, but unlike the latter there is no distinct fibrous capsule. On the other hand a central depressed scar as seen here is frequently present. Focal nodular hyperplasia is similar to benign adenoma in its relationship to steroid therapy with risk of serious bleeding.

10.4 Focal nodular hyperplasia ('focal cirrhosis')

Part of a small hamartoma is shown (lower right) including a portion of its central scar. Several fibrous septa radiate from the scar into the remainder of the lesion which is not encapsulated but blends with normal parenchyma in the upper part of the illustration. The hepatocyte component bears a close resemblance to normal liver cells apart from fatty change in this case. × 30 Hematoxylin and eosin.

10.5 Focal nodular hyperplasia

This is part of the central scar which contains numerous small blood vessels and bile ductules. The blood vessels on the left have disproportionately thick walls. In some cases they are more prominent than this and there may be arteriovenous fistulas. Chronic inflammatory cells are present throughout. × 47 Hematoxylin and eosin.

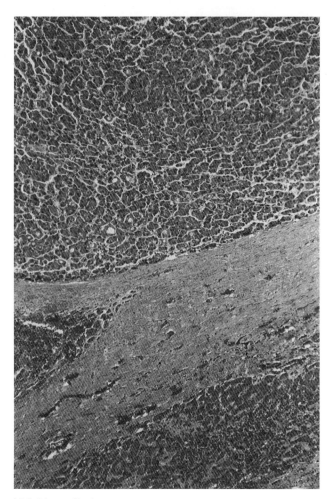

10.1 Liver cell adenoma.

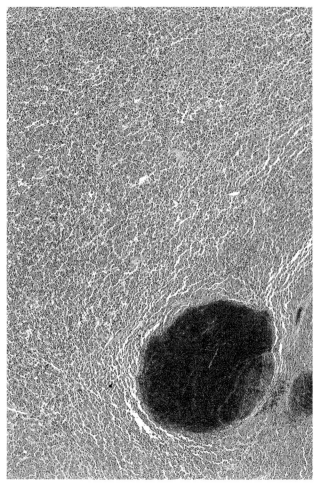

10.2 Liver cell adenoma.

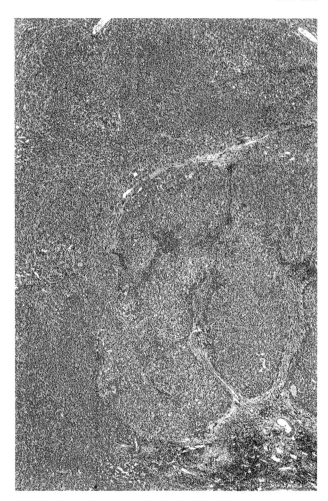

10.4 Focal nodular hyperplasia ('focal cirrhosis').

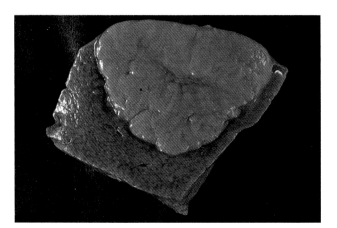

10.3 Focal nodular hyperplasia.

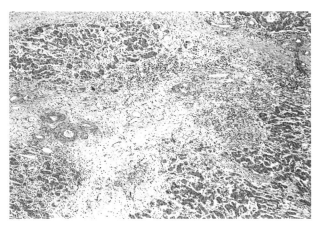

10.5 Focal nodular hyperplasia.

10.6 Hepatocellular carcinoma in non-cirrhotic liver

There is a large central tumour mass and a number of smaller satellite nodules. Parts of the tumour, especially in the centre of the field, show pale areas of necrosis but there is no umbilication of subcapsular nodules as in some cases of secondary carcinoma (**10.72**). Only a minority of these tumours arise in non-cirrhotic livers and not infrequently they consist of large solitary lesions.

10.7 Hepatocellular carcinoma in cirrhotic liver

Malignant change has occurred at multifocal sites producing nodules of variable size; these are much paler than the hyperplastic nodules of cirrhosis. Cirrhosis in this case is macronodular and was crypto-genic.

10.8 Hepatocellular carcinoma in cirrhotic liver

A case of micronodular alcoholic cirrhosis in which there are very numerous small pale foci of malignant change. Malignancy in alcoholic liver disease occurs more commonly in association with a coarser type of cirrhosis. It often follows a period of abstention from alcohol which permits better regenerative activity, but this would appear to promote neoplasia in some cases.

10.9 Hepatocellular carcinoma in cirrhotic liver

In this case of posthepatitis cirrhosis there is a small area of rather ill-defined malignancy to the right of the site of removal of a block of tissue for histological examination. This part is slightly elevated and less nodular than the surrounding liver.

10.10 Hepatocellular carcinoma in cirrhotic liver

The cut surface of the liver shown in **10.9** includes the small neoplastic pale area at the apex of the specimen. Such an early lesion may be missed if examination of cirrhotic liver is cursory.

10.11 Hepatocellular carcinoma: vascular invasion

This non-cirrhotic liver contained a large hepatocellular carcinoma which is imparting a nodular appearance to the upper surface of the right lobe (top right). These tumours tend to invade blood vessels and in this case a large nodule has grown through a hepatic venous ostium and partly fills the lumen of the inferior vena cava which is laid open.

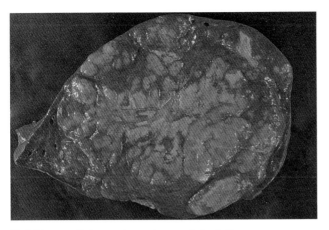

10.6 Hepatocellular carcinoma in non-cirrhotic liver.

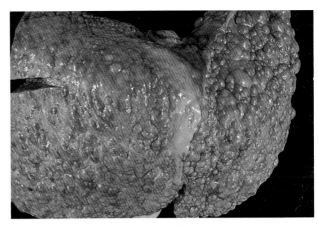

10.9 Hepatocellular carcinoma in cirrhotic liver.

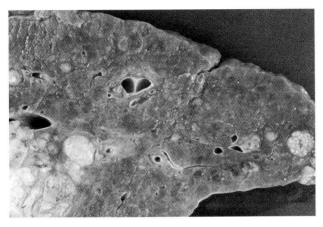

10.7 Hepatocellular carcinoma in cirrhotic liver.

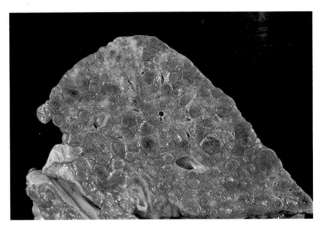

10.10 Hepatocellular carcinoma in cirrhotic liver.

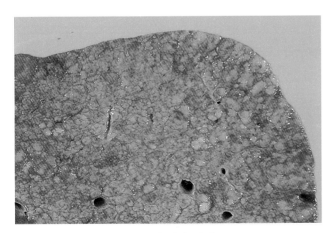

10.8 Hepatocellular carcinoma in cirrhotic liver.

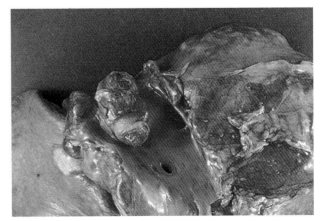

10.11 Hepatocellular carcinoma: vascular invasion.

10.12 Hepatocellular carcinoma

This photograph shows well-differentiated tumour cells. Many of those above are arranged in a trabecular fashion between narrow vascular sinusoids. Others (below) have an acinar or pseudoglandular arrangement around small channels which may act as capillaries for bile secreted by the tumour cells. Both these patterns are relatively common in hepatocellular carcinoma. Fibrous tissue is inconspicuous. × 117 Hematoxylin and eosin.

10.13 Hepatocellular carcinoma in cirrhotic liver

The tumour cells are arranged in groups separated by fibrous tissue and thus maintain the pre-existing cirrhotic pattern. Shrinkage of tumour nodules can give a false impression of vascular invasion. This mixture of neoplastic and non-neoplastic nodules is characteristic of certain primary liver cancers. × 47 Hematoxylin and eosin.

10.14 Hepatocellular carcinoma: fibrous stroma

Reticulin fibres in the nodule of hepatocellular carcinoma above are very fine and inconspicuous compared with those of normal liver (below). Nevertheless these tumours are capable of synthesizing collagen and prolyl hydroxylase, an enzyme related to this activity; indeed, high serum levels of the enzyme may be a useful diagnostic test. Presumably the tumour collagen is unstable or susceptible to collagenolytic factors which may be present also. × 146 Reticulin stain.

10.15 Hepatocellular carcinoma: invasion of adjacent liver

Nodules of primary liver cancer may remain discrete or invade adjacent tissue, as in the centre of this field. The tumour cells are hyperchromatic and pleomorphic but retain some resemblance to normal hepatocytes. Degeneration and loss of tumour cells in the centres of small groups produces a pseudoglandular appearance which is shown here. × 75 Hematoxylin and eosin.

10.16 Hepatocellular carcinoma: bile production

Plugs of green bile are prominent in this tumour and are a product of the cancer cells. Normal liver is present (bottom right). Discoloration of tumour by bile pigment may be seen on naked eye examination, especially after fixation. This phenomenon is specific for hepatocellular carcinoma but can be detected in only a minority of cases. × 75 Van Gieson's stain and hematoxylin.

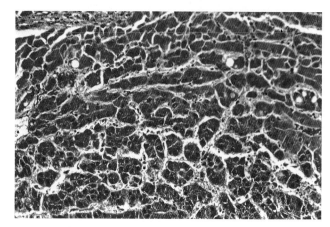

10.12 Hepatocellular carcinoma.

10.17 Hepatocellular carcinoma: acinar pattern

In some tumours an acinar pattern is the prominent histological feature. These channels often contain bile pigment which is unusually profuse in this case. They must not be confused with cholangiocarcinoma (**10.43**) which is scirrhous, consists of deeper-staining cells with less cytoplasm and does not synthesize bile. × 59 Hematoxylin and eosin.

10.18 Hepatocellular carcinoma: bile pigment in metastatic deposits

There are two metastatic deposits in the lung, one of which contains a plug of bile pigment within a tumour acinus (arrow). In less well differentiated tumours, the presence of bile provides conclusive evidence of histogenesis. Metastatic deposits are found most frequently in lymph nodes in the porta hepatis and in lung parenchyma, but are absent in at least half of all fatal cases. × 117 Hematoxylin and eosin.

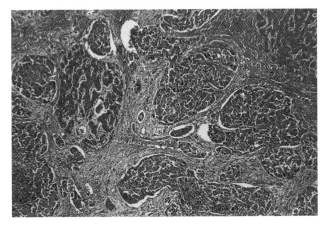

10.13 Hepatocellular carcinoma in cirrhotic liver.

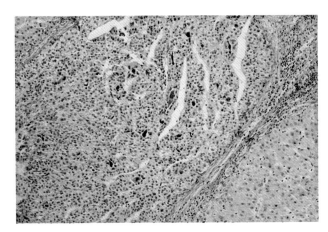

10.16 Hepatocellular carcinoma: bile production.

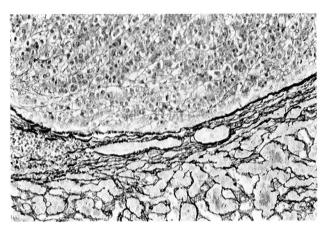

10.14 Hepatocellular carcinoma: fibrous stroma.

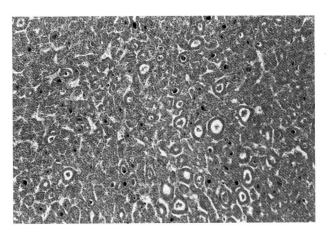

10.17 Hepatocellular carcinoma: acinar pattern.

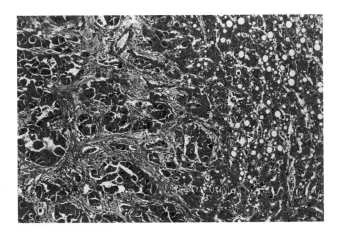

10.15 Hepatocellular carcinoma: invasion of adjacent liver.

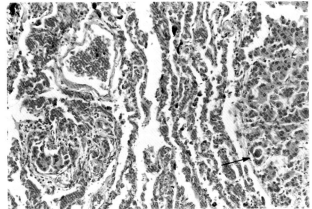

10.18 Hepatocellular carcinoma: bile pigment in metastatic deposits.

10.19 Hepatocellular carcinoma: cobblestone pattern

Rarely in some tumours or parts of tumour, cells of fairly uniform appearance form solid sheets which have been likened to cobblestone paving, and this is such an example. A few tiny acinar structures are seen but these are not an essential component of the lesion. There is a little fibro-vascular stroma in places. A resemblance to adrenal rest tumour (**10.70**) may be noted, but other portions of the specimen illustrated here showed bile synthesis, thus confirming its hepato-cellular origin. × 117 Hematoxylin and eosin.

10.20 Hepatocellular carcinoma: small-cell type

There is a nodule of tumour which abuts on normal hepatic tissue (below and on the left) with no inter-vening fibrous stroma. The tumour cells are small and stain deeply although their cytoplasm appears vacuo-lated, probably due to lipid or glycogen. Vacuolation is sometimes very prominent ('clear cell' liver cancer). These small cell tumours can be difficult to diagnose but the trabecular pattern in this example is suggestive of a liver cell origin. It is important if possible to examine several blocks of tissue from such a specimen, since other portions of the tumour can be more characteristic of hepatocellular carcinoma. × 75 Hematoxylin and eosin.

10.21 Hepatocellular carcinoma: giant-cell type

Some parts of this tumour, which occupies the entire field, are necrotic while others survive as multi-nucleated syncytial masses. The pleomorphism and lack of an orderly pattern of cell arrangement make the diagnosis of these tumours difficult but, as with the small-cell variety, other parts often show a more orderly arrangement of cells into trabecular and acinar structures which are more typical of primary liver cancer. × 71 Hematoxylin and eosin.

10.22 Hepatocellular carcinoma: glycogen in tumour cells

This is a small cell primary liver cancer with glycogen in the cytoplasm giving positive PAS-staining which would be prevented by pretreatment with diastase. More intense glycogen staining is given by the narrow band of surviving non-malignant hepatocytes (right). The presence of glycogen in the tumour may help to establish its liver origin, but the test is not specific since other cancers which may be confused with hepatocellular tumours, especially renal and adrenal cortical cancers, sometimes contain glycogen. × 117 Periodic acid-Schiff method and hematoxylin.

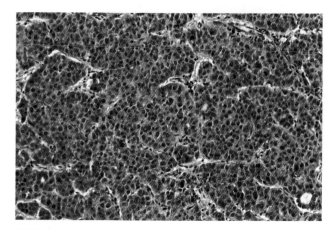

10.19 Hepatocellular carcinoma: cobblestone pattern.

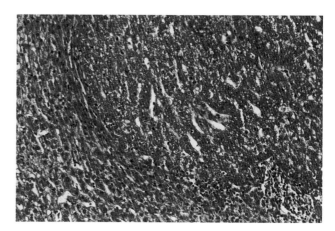

10.20 Hepatocellular carcinoma: small-cell type.

10.23 Hepatocellular carcinoma: lipid in tumour cells

A portion of tumour in which many of the cells contain large lipid droplets. The amount of both lipid and glycogen in primary liver cancer cells is very variable and fat was not seen in other tumour nodules from this specimen. × 117 Hematoxylin and eosin.

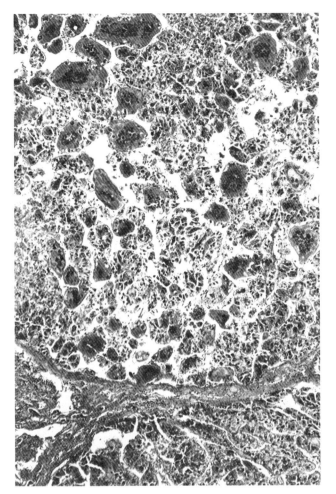

10.21 Hepatocellular carcinoma: giant-cell type.

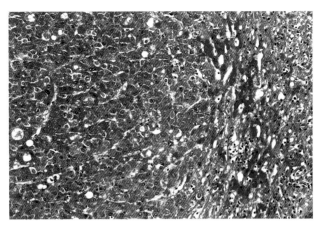

10.22 Hepatocellular carcinoma: glycogen in tumour cells.

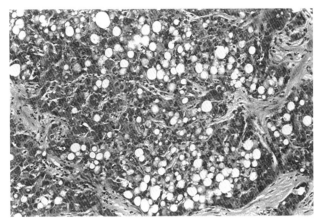

10.23 Hepatocellular carcinoma: lipid in tumour cells.

10.24 Hepatocellular carcinoma: hyaline degeneration

This field consists entirely of hepatocellular cancer. Mallory bodies are present in several tumour cells (arrows). This unusual feature of liver-cell carcinoma is commonly associated with chronic alcoholism. In this case the tumour had arisen as a complication of alcoholic cirrhosis. × 234 Hematoxylin and eosin.

10.25 Hepatocellular carcinoma: hyaline inclusion bodies

Numerous globular eosinophilic bodies are present in this tumour. Many are located in the cell cytoplasm and some are sharply defined. They are presumably a product of cancer cell metabolism such as α-feto-protein, but could not be further characterized in this case. × 187 Hematoxylin and eosin.

10.26 Hepatocellular carcinoma: hyaline inclusion bodies

The same specimen as shown in **10.25** stained by the PAS technique after diastase treatment. Failure to stain inclusion bodies indicates that they are not α1-antitrypsin. Abundant cell cytoplasm and prominent nucleoli are characteristic features of hepatocellular cancer. × 281 Periodic acid-Schiff method and hematoxylin.

10.27 Hepatocellular carcinoma: α1-antitrypsin inclusions

A few liver-cell cancers contain inclusions of this protein which are PAS-positive and diastase-resistant. In this case their true nature was confirmed immuno-histochemically. Persons with α1-antitrypsin deficiency have a higher than normal incidence of primary liver-cell cancer. × 234 Periodic acid-Schiff method and hematoxylin.

10.28 Hepatocellular carcinoma: hepatitis B infection of liver

This section of cirrhotic liver shows part of a nodule of primary liver cancer (top left). Many hepatocytes , right,give positive cytoplasmic staining for hepatitis B surface antigen by the immunoperoxidase technique (**6.25**). Evidence for this association of infection and tumour is found in most countries and is strong in places such as East Africa where the incidence of primary liver cancer is high. Positive staining for the hepatitis B surface antigen is found usually in the non-neoplastic liver cells but it can occur in tumour cells. This association may be independent of the presence of cirrhosis. × 45 Immunoperoxidase.

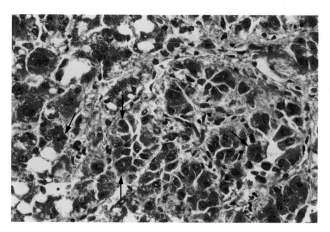

10.24 Hepatocellular carcinoma: hyaline degeneration.

10.29 Hepatocellular carcinoma: hepatitis B infection of liver

These are photographs of a fairly well differentiated hepatocellular carcinoma. That on the right illustrates that many tumour cells have positive cytoplasmic staining for hepatitis B surface antigen as shown by the immunoperoxidase technique. The control section on the left gives negative staining with serum in which the hepatitis surface antibody had been absorbed with its appropriate antigen. × 187 Immunoperoxidase.

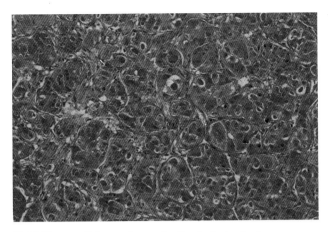

10.25 Hepatocellular carcinoma: hyaline inclusion bodies.

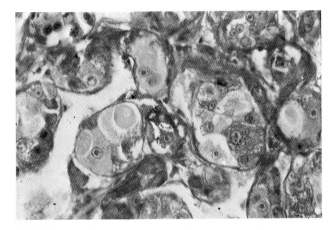

10.26 Hepatocellular carcinoma: hyaline inclusion bodies.

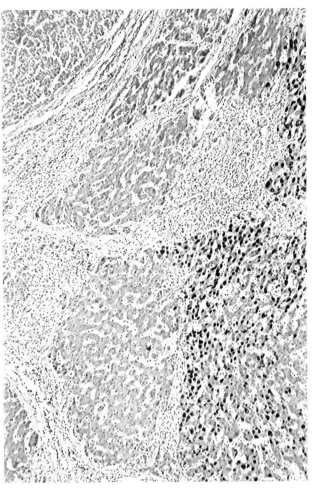

10.28 Hepatocellular carcinoma: hepatitis B infection of liver.

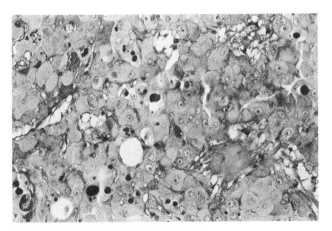

10.27 Hepatocellular carcinoma: α1-antitrypsin inclusions.

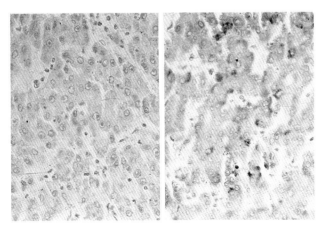

10.29 Hepatocellular carcinoma: hepatitis B infection of liver.

10.30 Hepatocellular carcinoma: hemochromatosis

Patients with hemochromatosis appear to have a tendency to primary liver cancer. It is possible, however, that the association is between cancer and the cirrhosis induced by excessive amounts of hemosiderin in the liver, rather than a more direct one between cancer and hemosiderin. In this field iron-containing pigment in non-neoplastic hepatocytes gives a strongly positive Prussian blue reaction. By contrast the tumour nodules, in which some cancer cells are forming small acini, do not contain pigment. × 30 Perls' method and neutral red.

10.31 Hepatocellular carcinoma: vascularity

This is an example of an excessively vascular tumour which could cause severe or even fatal intra-abdominal bleeding. These cases should not be mistaken for angiosarcoma, but the tumour cells are fairly typical of primary liver-cell cancer. Unusual vascularity such as this may be associated with prolonged anabolic and androgenic steroid therapy. × 47 Hematoxylin and eosin.

10.32 Hepatocellular carcinoma: vascular invasion

Hepatocellular carcinoma has a distinct tendency to invade portal and hepatic venous channels and lymphatics within the liver, and this can contribute to portal hypertension. Direct extension of tumour along hepatic veins to inferior vena cava is possible. This section shows cancer cells and fibrin within a dilated portal vein in the centre of the field. × 45 Hematoxylin and eosin.

10.33 Hepatocellular carcinoma: bile duct invasion

The photograph shows part of a grossly distended intrahepatic bile duct. The columnar epithelium lining the duct is preserved and runs across the centre of the field (above). The lumen contains a large clump of rather degenerate and partly necrotic primary liver cancer which had originated in the right lobe of the liver. Fragments of tumour were present also in the common bile duct and the patient's illness began as an obstructive-type jaundice. This is an unusual cause of cholestatic jaundice but several cases have been reported. × 71 Hematoxylin and eosin.

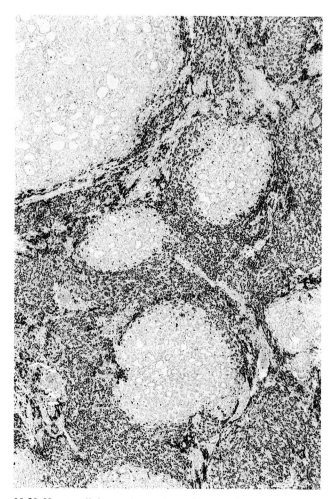

10.30 Hepatocellular carcinoma: hemochromatosis.

10.34 Hepatocellular carcinoma: invasion of nerve

Hepatocellular carcinoma in the region of the porta hepatis has a tendency to invade nerves. In this specimen well-differentiated liver-cell cancer is mainly perineural in distribution. × 47 Hematoxylin and eosin.

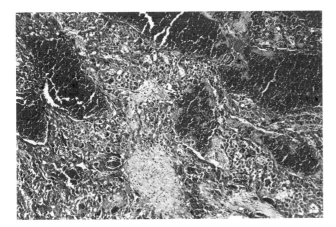

10.31 Hepatocellular carcinoma: vascularity.

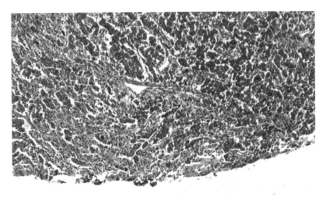

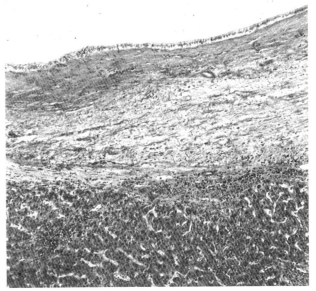

10.33 Hepatocellular carcinoma: bile duct invasion.

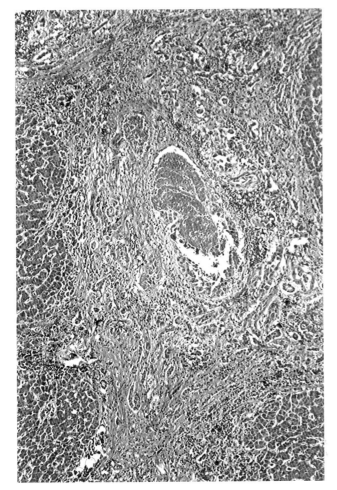

10.32 Hepatocellular carcinoma: vascular invasion.

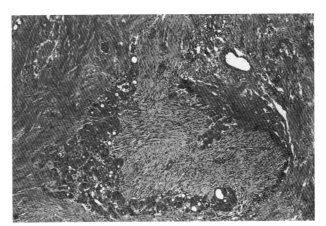

10.34 Hepatocellular carcinoma: invasion of nerve.

10.35 Hepatocellular carcinoma caused by thorotrast

Hepatocellular cancer is shown (top right and left and within a small vessel). To the left of the vessel are several small deposits of dull grey finely granular material (arrows) which is thorotrast administered about thirty years before the patient's death. Cholangiocarcinoma and angiosarcoma of liver may also arise in patients given this radioactive diagnostic agent. × 117 Hematoxylin and eosin.

10.36 Thorotrast in liver

Apart from the induction of malignancy, thorotrast causes portal and septal fibrosis. This photograph shows dark deposits of the material in fibrous portal tracts. A similar pattern of fibrosis may be induced by arsenical compounds and vinyl chloride which, like thorotrast, are also carcinogenic. × 47 Hematoxylin and eosin.

10.37 Thorotrast in liver

The presence of this material can be confirmed by autoradiography of paraffin sections as this detects its continuing radioactivity. Radioactivity is shown here by short black lines in the photographic emulsion which overlies the tumour section. Because of the thickness of the emulsion it is not possible to bring the underlying section into focus with the lines, but a deposit of thorotrast can be seen indistinctly in the centre of the field. × 234 Autoradiograph.

10.38 Liver-cell dysplasia

Part of a cirrhotic liver in which the smaller collection of hepatocytes (upper left) is of normal morphology. The remainder consists of larger cells with abundant eosinophilic cytoplasm and with nuclear pleomorphism and hyperchromatism. The significance of this dysplastic change is uncertain, but it appears to be associated with primary liver cancer in areas such as East Africa where the incidence of tumour is high. Hepatic dysplasia occurs also in experimental animals fed agents which induce liver-cell tumours. However, in the experimental type the nuclei of the affected cells tend to be enlarged and the cytoplasm basophilic. × 117 Hematoxylin and eosin.

10.39 Bile ductular adenoma

There is a non-encapsulated tumour immediately beneath the liver capsule (top left). It consists of small glandular structures with the morphology of bile ductules. These small white subcapsular tumours are found not infrequently but have no clinical significance. × 71 Hematoxylin and eosin.

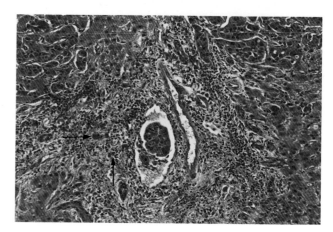

10.35 Hepatocellular carcinoma caused by thorotrast.

10.40 Intraduct biliary papilloma

A large distended septal bile duct has a focus of papillary epithelial proliferation. The degree of cellular pleomorphism is very suggestive of malignancy but such tumours can grow to produce obstructive jaundice without much evidence of invasion of surrounding tissue. In this case there was a second larger tumour causing biliary obstruction at the porta hepatis. It is probably best to regard these as papillary cancers of low-grade malignancy. Truly benign bile duct papillomas are probably very rare. × 117 Hematoxylin and eosin.

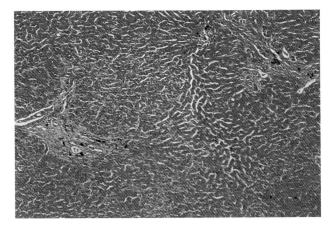

10.36 Thorotrast in liver.

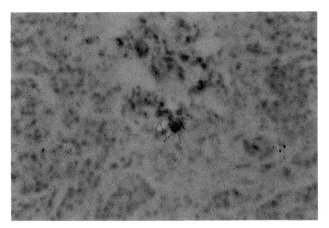

10.37 Thorotrast in liver.

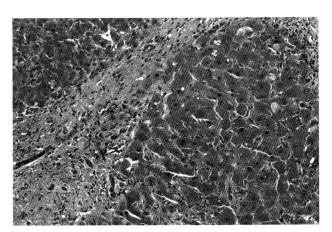

10.38 Liver-cell dysplasia.

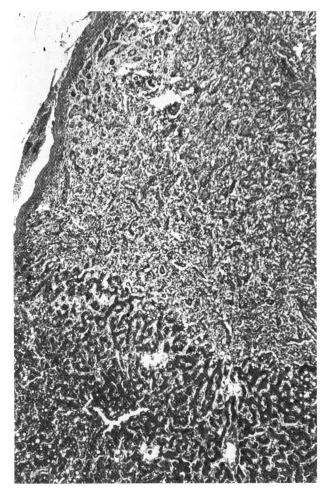

10.39 Bile ductular adenoma.

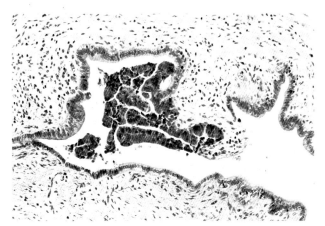

10.40 Intraduct biliary papilloma.

10.41 Cholangiocarcinoma of liver

The large brown tumour which had arisen in the region of the porta hepatis is spreading into the substance of the liver. There are a number of small satellite deposits and invasion of a large intrahepatic vein (lower centre). A few white areas of necrosis are seen. These tumours are never bile-stained and the intense green bile discoloration which is present here is confined to the surviving liver parenchyma and caused by obstruction to the outward flow of bile by the tumour at the porta hepatis.

10.42 Cholangiocarcinoma

This is taken near the site of origin of the tumour in a large duct situated within the liver. The epithelial lining of the stellate lumen is not neoplastic but there is hyperplasia and neoplasia of surrounding ducts. Neoplastic change is more obvious at the periphery where there are small glandular structures with distended lumens lined by deeply staining malignant epithelium. The stroma is rather scirrhous. Hyperplastic and dysplastic changes in bile duct epithelium are often seen in the vicinity of such tumours. × 30 Hematoxylin and eosin.

10.43 Cholangiocarcinoma

This shows the typically scirrhous nature of these tumours. There are a number of ductular structures of variable size lined by cuboidal or flattened cancer cells, some of which form small blunt papillae. × 52 Hematoxylin and eosin.

10.44 Cholangiocarcinoma

There was a tumour in the porta hepatis arising from the right hepatic duct and spreading distally within the liver especially in portal tracts. This shows part of a distal tumour nodule above, which consists of scirrhous adenocarcinoma. Lymphocytes are present at the margin of tumour and liver parenchyma below. Cholestasis is prominent because of obstruction to bile flow by the primary cancer. × 117 Hematoxylin and eosin.

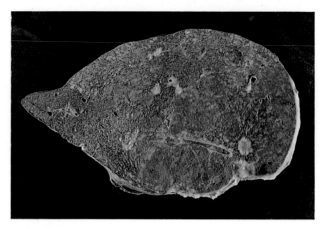

10.41 Cholangiocarcinoma of liver.

10.45 Cystadenocarcinoma of bile duct

An unusual tumour consisting of groups of acini lined by cuboidal epithelium and separated by a thin vascular stroma. There is a tendency to papilloma formation within distended acini. This was part of the thick wall of a mucin-containing cystic tumour arising from an intrahepatic duct. × 91 Hematoxylin and eosin.

10.46 Cholangiolocellular carcinoma

This uncommon tumour consists of small tubular structures like bile ductules lined by cuboidal epithelium. In places the tumour cells are arranged in two parallel rows without a distinct lumen. The fibrous stroma is conspicuous. × 117 Hematoxylin and eosin.

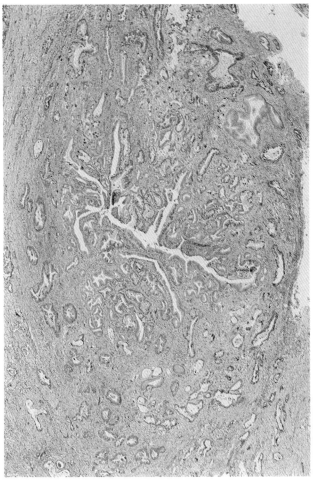

10.42 Cholangiocarcinoma.

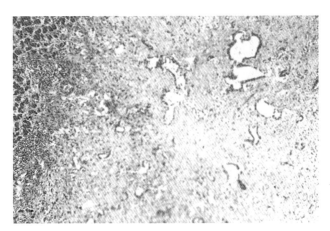

10.43 Cholangiocarcinoma.

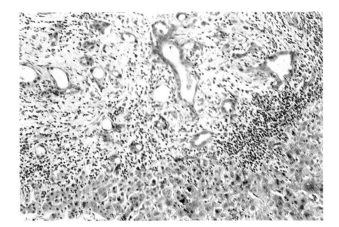

10.44 Cholangiocarcinoma.

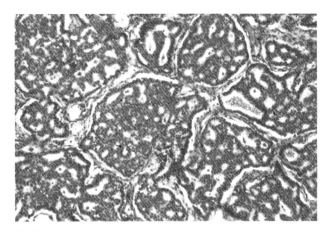

10.45 Cystadenocarcinoma of bile duct.

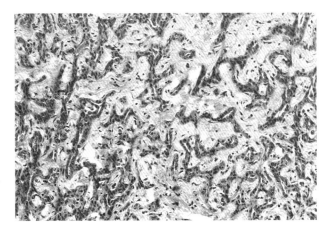

10.46 Cholangiolocellular carcinoma.

10.47 Mixed hepatocellular and cholangiocellular carcinoma

Cancer cells in the upper part of the field clearly resemble hepatocytes, and there was some evidence of bile production in this part. In the lower part they are smaller and are forming small acinar structures set in a fibrous stroma as seen in typical bile duct cancer. This liver contained numerous tumour deposits of variable size which consisted of one or other of these cell types. It has been suggested that malignancy originates independently in hepatocytes and bile duct epithelium and that the two tumours develop together, retaining their individual characteristics. × 59 Hematoxylin and eosin.

10.48 Transitional hepatocellular and cholangiocellular carcinoma

This field showing adenocarcinoma was typical of the tumour as a whole. It consists of cells which appear to be transitional between hepatocytes and bile duct epithelium. Both mixed and transitional types of primary liver cancer are uncommon. × 75 Hematoxylin and eosin.

10.49 Bile ductular proliferation in hepatocellular carcinoma

A small-cell primary liver cancer is present (top left). The remainder of the photograph shows a scirrhous area with a few surviving hepatocytes (below) and much bile ductular proliferation. Bile ductular proliferation occurs not uncommonly in association with hepatocellular carcinoma. It should not be mistaken for the bile duct cancer component of a mixed tumour. × 71 Hematoxylin and eosin.

10.50 Bile ductular proliferation in hepatocellular carcinoma

Another example of this phenomenon occurring in a primary hepatocellular carcinoma, a small part of which is shown on the left. Much of the fibrous stroma of the tumour contains numerous small bile ducts and ductules. × 117 Hematoxylin and eosin.

10.51 Primary liver cancer (experimental)

A rat fed a riboflavine-deficient diet with the addition of p-dimethylaminoazobenzine (DAB) for twenty weeks. The liver is enormously enlarged and nodular and histological examination confirmed the presence of primary carcinoma. Despite the large size of the tumour, metastatic deposits were not present.

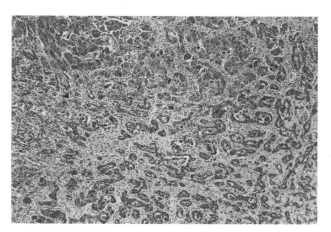

10.47 Mixed hepatocellular and cholangiocellular carcinoma.

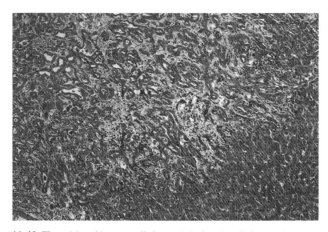

10.48 Transitional hepatocellular and cholangiocellular carcinoma.

10.52 Primary liver cancer (experimental)

Many tumours produced experimentally with DAB are of mixed histological type. All epithelial cells in this field are neoplastic; those left of centre constitute hepatocellular carcinoma while those on the right form cystic cholangiocarcinoma with a little mucus secretion. The remainder have transitional features. × 117 Hematoxylin and eosin.

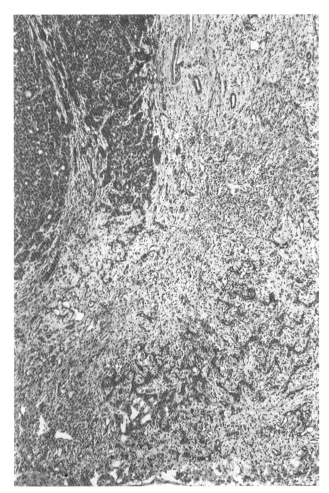

10.49 Bile ductular proliferation in hepatocellular carcinoma.

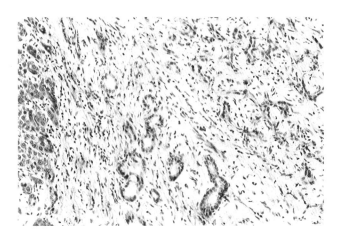

10.50 Bile ductular proliferation in hepatocellular carcinoma.

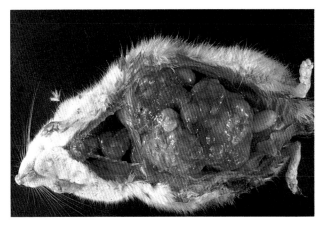

10.51 Primary liver cancer (experimental).

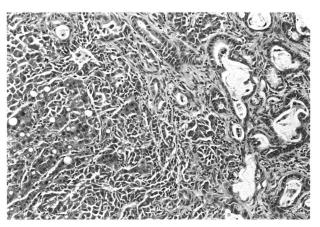

10.52 Primary liver cancer (experimental).

10.53 Cavernous hemangioma of liver

These tumours are usually small and situated just under the capsule as shown in this figure. Occasionally they are much larger especially in young children when they may be complicated by microangiopathic hemolytic anemia, high-output cardiac failure or serious intra-abdominal bleeding. Some are multiple and this may indicate involvement of the liver in multiple telangiectasia syndrome (Chapter 3).

10.54 Cavernous hemangioma

This shows the histological appearance of a typical example. It consists of blood-filled cystic spaces lined by flattened endothelium and separated by thin bands of fibrous tissue. Its situation under Glisson's capsule is evident, but there is no fibrous capsule separating it from normal liver parenchyma below. These are very common lesions and most are symptomless. They may undergo thrombosis and fibrosis, sometimes with calcification. × 36 Hematoxylin and eosin.

10.55 Cavernous hemangioma: hematopoiesis

Foci of dark-staining hematopoietic tissue are present in the spaces of this cavernous angioma. A similar phenomenon can occur in hemangioendothelioma and angiosarcoma. This is an uncommon finding in these tumours except in young children. This specimen was from an adult with no evidence of hematopoiesis elsewhere and no bone marrow disease. × 71 Hematoxylin and eosin.

10.56 Hemangioendothelioma of liver

This is part of a very large tumour in the liver of a woman aged 45 which had grown over a period of several years to occupy much of the right lobe. It consists of irregularly shaped endothelium-lined spaces, some of which contain a little blood. These are separated by a fibrous stroma and portions of the infiltrated liver which survive as small nodules of parenchyma and bile ducts. Several biopsies of this lesion presented a similar appearance of what appears to be primarily a vascular tumour. Hemangioendothelioma is very uncommon in adults. × 71 Hematoxylin and eosin.

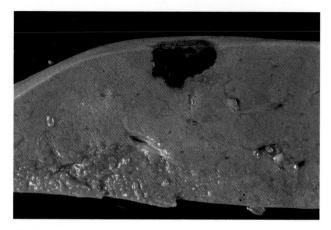

10.53 Cavernous hemangioma of liver.

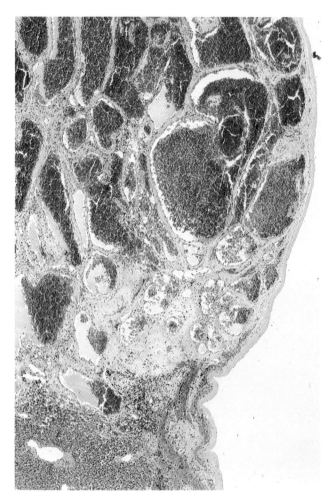

10.54 Cavernous hemangioma.

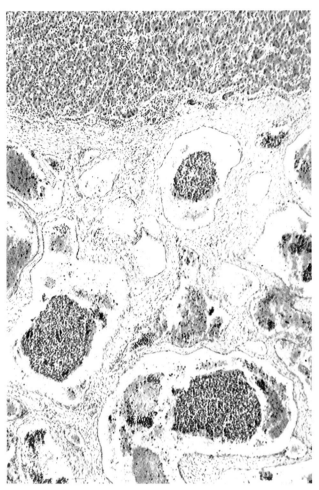

10.55 Cavernous hemangioma: hematopoiesis.

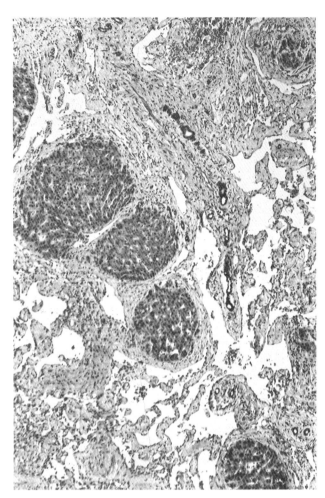

10.56 Hemangioendothelioma of liver.

10.57 Hemangioendothelioma of liver

The tumour consists mostly of endothelium, the cells forming solid masses or small vascular structures. Such lesions are usually found in young infants and may grow to a very large size. They are non-invasive but death may occur from atrophy and compression of the liver, or from cardiac failure which can be mistaken for primary congenital heart disease. In those patients who survive, the condition undergoes regression with fibrosis. × 187 Hematoxylin and eosin.

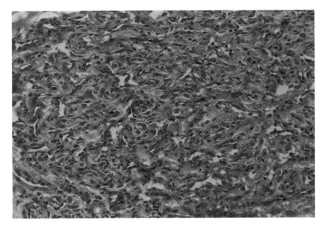

10.57 Hemangioendothelioma of liver.

10.58 Angiosarcoma of liver

A section through liver and gallbladder shows wide-spread involvement of the former by blood-containing tumour deposits. The largest on the left forms a multiloculated cystic structure which was filled with clotted blood. The patient had a five-month history of liver disease and died of intra-abdominal bleeding. There were no metastatic deposits in this case.

10.59 Angiosarcoma of liver

Another portion of the liver shown in **10.58**. Here the tumour deposits are smaller and there is much surviving non-cirrhotic liver. Some cases of angio-sarcoma do arise in cirrhotic liver. Some can be attributed to ingestion of vinyl chloride, arsenical compounds or thorotrast, but the etiology of this case was not discovered.

10.60 Angiosarcoma of liver

In this field many tumour cells appear as endothelium lining blood filled spaces not unlike benign cavernous hemangioma. However, compared with normal endo-thelium these lining cells are hyperchromatic and, in the upper part, they are showing some tendency to heap up and form multinucleated syncytial struc-tures. The invasive nature of the tumour is also apparent in this upper part where there are a few surviving hepatocytes surrounded by vascular spaces. ×130 Hematoxylin and eosin.

10.61 Angiosarcoma of liver

On the left tumour replaces hepatic parenchyma. The sarcoma cells have hyperchromatic nuclei which are spindle-shaped or pleomorphic. On the right tumour helps to line sinusoids between surviving cords of hepatocytes. ×117 Hematoxylin and eosin.

10.62 Angiosarcoma of liver

Hyperchromatic tumour cells line small portions of surviving liver cell cords and even individual hepato-cytes. The intervening spaces contain blood. This isolation of viable liver cells by tumour is rather characteristic of angiosarcoma. ×187 Hematoxylin and eosin.

10.63 Angiosarcoma of liver

A solid area of tumour cells many of which are rounded while others are flattened and line very in-distinct channels. The appearances are not unlike hemangioendothelioma (**10.57**) but there is more cellular pleomorphism and hyperchromatism. While the interpretation of such a field can be difficult, examination of other parts of the tumour usually reveals features more characteristic of its true nature. ×234 Hematoxylin and eosin.

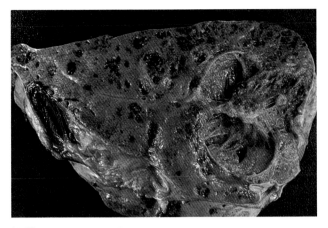

10.58 Angiosarcoma of liver.

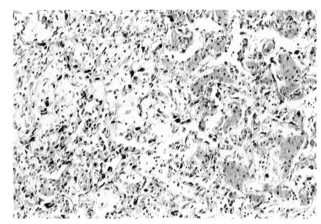

10.61 Angiosarcoma of liver.

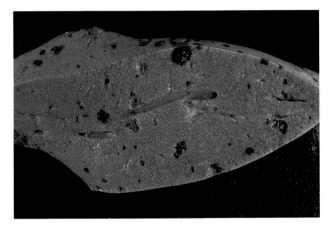

10.59 Angiosarcoma of liver.

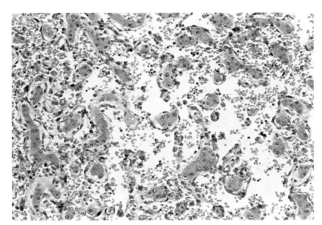

10.62 Angiosarcoma of liver.

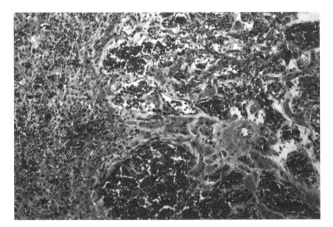

10.60 Angiosarcoma of liver.

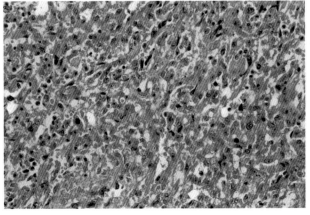

10.63 Angiosarcoma of liver.

10.64 Hepatoblastoma

The deeply-stained parts of this tumour consist of fetal liver parenchyma which closely resembles normal infantile hepatic tissue. A nodule of pale primitive mesenchyme which is an inherent component of the lesion, is seen. Below and to the right there is a band of denser more mature fibrous tissue, part of a fibrous septum which traversed the tumour. These are rare tumours occurring in infancy. They grow quickly and are usually fatal because of liver destruction, metastatic deposits or rupture with intraperitoneal bleeding, but successful resection is possible. The epithelial component is always present but the amount of mesenchyme varies considerably from case to case and may be difficult to find. × 47 Hematoxylin and eosin.

10.65 Hepatoblastoma

A narrow band of fetal-type liver runs diagonally from above downwards and to the right (arrows). A collection of embryonic-type hepatocytes is present on the left; these are more markedly hyperchromatic and tend to form tubular structures or rosettes. The degree of malignancy is highest in the embryonic component of hepatoblastoma, but embryonic cells are not found in all cases. The cells of the fetal component may resemble normal infant hepatocytes closely and often contain some glycogen and fat. Collections of hemopoietic cells may be prominent in those parts of the tumour which consists of fetal cells. Areas of hemorrhage and necrosis may be extensive. × 146 Hematoxylin and eosin.

10.66 Hepatoblastoma

This field shows an island of osteoid tissue surrounded by the epithelial component of the tumour. Osteoid is present in only a minority of cases, the mesenchymal component usually consisting of poorly differentiated fibrous connective tissue as seen in **10.64**. Cartilage is very uncommon. × 47 Hematoxylin and eosin.

10.67 Rhabdomyosarcoma of liver

Part of the tumour found at post-mortem examination of a five-year-old child. The tumour occupied most of the liver. The majority of cells are small and rounded but some are spindle-shaped and there is a scattering of giant forms. The appearances were uniform throughout the tumour and are characteristic of embryonal rhabdomyosarcoma. These uncommon tumours affect young children but of a somewhat older age group compared with hepatoblastoma. The two types of tumour are distinct, and skeletal muscle is not a component of hepatoblastoma. Poorly-formed bile ductular structures may be found in rhabdomyosarcoma but were not detected in this case. Neither were there any cells with cross-striations but these are hardly ever seen in embryonal tumours. It is suggested that a non-adult form of rhabdomyosarcoma can develop in the liver from the wall of large bile ducts and that these may contain cells with cross-striations. × 113 Hematoxylin and eosin.

10.68 Spindle-cell tumours in liver

Tumours such as benign and malignant smooth-muscle neoplasms have been described, some of which may arise from the walls of blood vessels or ligamentum teres. More commonly they are sarcomatous metastatic deposits from an extrahepatic primary lesion such as this example of secondary leiomyosarcoma which arose in the stomach. Fibrosarcoma and malignant schwannoma have been reported as arising within the liver, but both are very rare. The former may be associated with the occurrence of hypoglycemia. × 75 Hematoxylin and eosin.

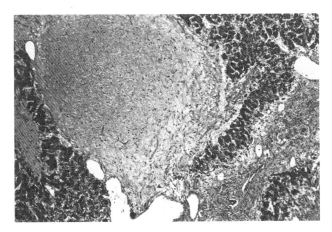

10.64 Hepatoblastoma.

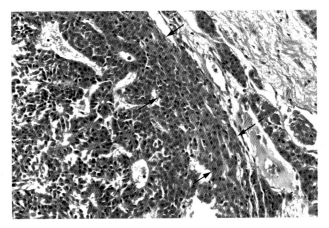

10.65 Hepatoblastoma.

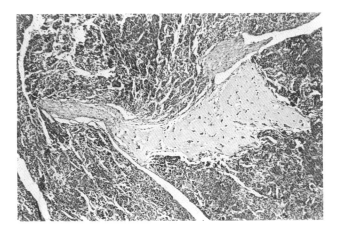

10.66 Hepatoblastoma.

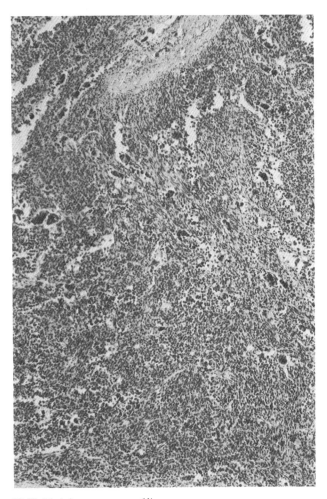

10.67 Rhabdomyosarcoma of liver.

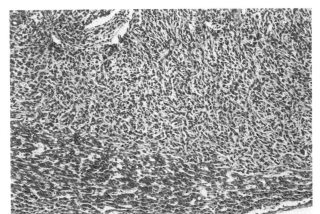

10.68 Spindle-cell tumours in liver.

10.69 Adrenal-rest tumour

Part of the nodular lesion is seen under the liver capsule. It was found in the right hepatic lobe adjacent to the inferior vena cava. It represents a rest of adrenal cortical tissue in which neoplastic change had occurred. No normal right adrenal gland was found at autopsy. There was no sign of primary carcinoma arising in the right kidney or elsewhere in the body. ×6 Hematoxylin and eosin.

10.70 Adrenal-rest tumour

A higher magnification of the tumour illustrated in **10.69**. Some of these cases may be mistaken for hepatocellular cancer, but they do not have a trabecular arrangement of cells along elongated sinusoids. By contrast the cells tend to form spherical clusters separated by a fine vascular stroma. Small acinar structures or rosettes may be seen within these clusters. Some adrenal rest tumours are hormonally active. ×75 Hematoxylin and eosin.

10.71 Secondary carcinoma: solitary lesion

This shows the cut surface of a bisected partial hepatectomy specimen containing a large single deposit of secondary carcinoma. The primary cancer in colon was also resected successfully and the patient made a good recovery with no recurrence of tumour over several years. Occasional cases of carcinoma especially from colon, kidney or an endocrine gland produce a single secondary hepatic deposit which can be treated in this way.

10.72 Secondary carcinoma: umbilication

There are numerous pale secondary deposits of tumour, many with a central depression due to ischemic necrosis. In cachectic patients this phenomenon of 'umbilication' of large tumour deposits can be palpated through a wasted anterior abdominal wall. Umbilication is unusual in primary liver cell cancer (**10.6**). In this case the primary tumour was in stomach, but it is rarely possible to assess the origin from gross appearance alone.

10.73 Secondary carcinoma: ischemic necrosis

Central ischemic necrosis is seen in several nodules of secondary bronchial cancer within the liver.

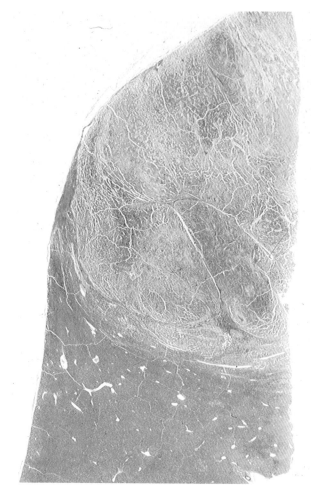

10.69 Adrenal-rest tumour.

10.74 Secondary carcinoma in cirrhotic liver

This is an infrequent finding although conflicting opinions have been expressed on the true incidence. In this case of cryptogenic macronodular cirrhosis the deposits of cancer were derived from a primary tumour in stomach. The clinical history suggested the presence of established cirrhosis for a number of years prior to the onset of gastric neoplasm.

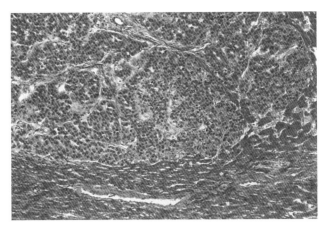

10.70 Adrenal-rest tumour.

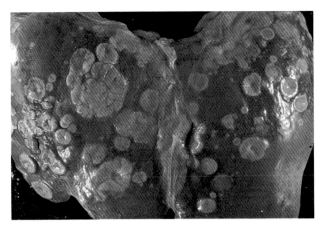

10.72 Secondary carcinoma: umbilication.

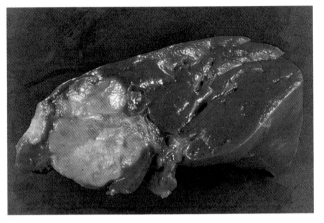

10.71 Secondary carcinoma: solitary lesion.

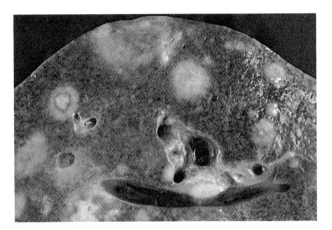

10.73 Secondary carcinoma: ischemic necrosis.

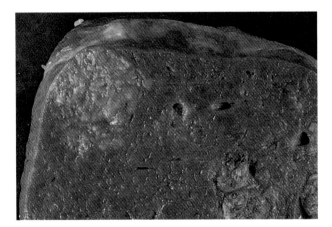

10.74 Secondary carcinoma in cirrhotic liver.

10.75 Secondary carcinoma: diffuse infiltration

Part of a greatly enlarged liver from a patient with primary breast cancer. The tumour forms nodules of various sizes, many being no larger than white pinpoints. In addition the normal markings of surviving parenchyma are lost because of diffuse sinusoidal infiltration by cancer which was confirmed by histological examination. Fibrosis sometimes develops round metastatic deposits. When there is extensive infiltration of the liver by tumour which possesses this characteristic, a form of diffuse fibrosis or cirrhosis may develop and cause portal hypertension, so-called 'carcinomatous cirrhosis'.

10.76 Secondary malignant melanoma: diffuse infiltration

Many sinusoids contain groups or columns of pigmented tumour cells but there is survival of most hepatocytes. The liver was greatly enlarged and black in colour. × 117 Hematoxylin and eosin.

10.77 Secondary carcinoma: microdeposits

In some liver biopsies secondary cancer may be confined to single cells or small groups lying in sinusoids or larger blood vessels. Here a small group of colonic cancer cells lies within a portal vein. × 117 Hematoxylin and eosin.

10.78 Secondary carcinoma: calcification

This shows part of a large deposit of adenocarcinoma which contains numerous small black granules of calcium salts. Calcification is a feature of some colonic cancer deposits of which this is an example, and may be detected radiologically. × 47 Hematoxylin and eosin.

10.79 Secondary carcinoma: hemorrhage

Deposits of carcinoma from a primary pancreatic tumour are delineated by cuffs of recent hemorrhage. This is a feature of some of these tumours and may be due to secretion of active pancreatic enzymes. × 47 Hematoxylin and eosin.

10.80 Secondary carcinoid tumour of liver

The histogenesis of certain malignant deposits may be assessed by their distinct morphology and staining, such as this example of carcinoid tumour giving a positive diazo reaction. The primary tumour was in the small intestine. Rare cases of carcinoid are described which arise within the liver, possibly from argentaffin cells in the walls of larger bile ducts. × 117 Diazo method for argentaffin cell granules and hematoxylin.

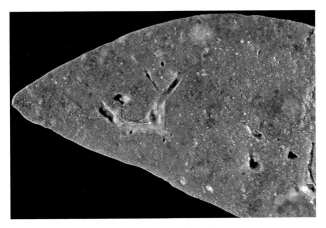

10.75 Secondary carcinoma: diffuse infiltration.

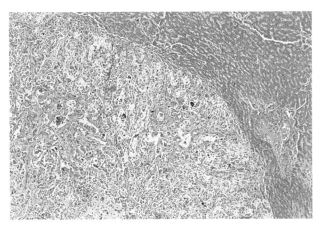

10.78 Secondary carcinoma: calcification.

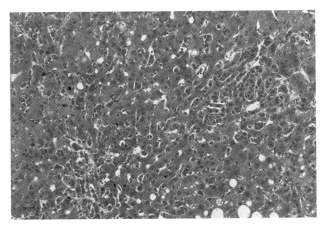

10.76 Secondary malignant melanoma: diffuse infiltration.

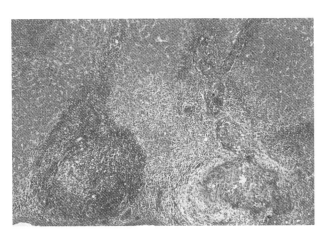

10.79 Secondary carcinoma: hemorrhage.

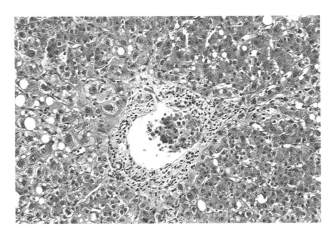

10.77 Secondary carcinoma: microdeposits.

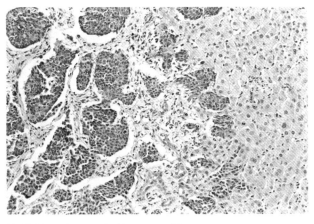

10.80 Secondary carcinoid tumour of liver.

10.81 Lymphosarcoma involving liver

A tumour of small lymphocyte type which is forming a dense collection of cells, especially in portal tracts where persistent bile ducts are seen. The uniform appearance of tumour cells helps to distinguish small deposits of this nature from chronic inflammatory lesions in portal tracts, especially in primary biliary cirrhosis. × 71 Hematoxylin and eosin.

10.82 Liver in leukemia

In this case of prolymphocytic leukemia portal infiltration with tumour cells resembles that seen in lymphosarcoma (**10.81**). In addition many dark staining leukemic cells form narrow columns within sinusoids. × 117 Hematoxylin and eosin.

10.83 Liver in leukemia

In this case of chronic myeloid leukemia the sinusoids are infiltrated diffusely with leukemic cells, some of which assume an Indian file pattern. The uniform involvement of liver helps to distinguish leukemia from conditions such as septicemia with leukocytosis and Kupffer cell hyperplasia, and from hematopoiesis which is most marked in the portal areas. The liver in 'big spleen disease' (tropical splenomegaly, **8.21**) may resemble lymphatic leukemia and some so-called 'non-tropical' cases may be examples of hairy cell leukemia. The latter condition can cause focal sinusoidal dilatation resembling peliosis hepatis. × 146 Hematoxylin and eosin.

10.84 Liver in leukemia

This illustrates hairy cell leukemia in liver. The leukemic cells have dark round or oval nuclei and their cytoplasmic borders may be irregular in shape or poorly defined. Many are lying free within sinusoids but a few appear to act as a sinusoidal lining. Sinusoidal dilatation may occur (upper right). The presence of this disease may first come to light in liver biopsy specimens. × 585 Hematoxylin and eosin.

10.85 Liver in Hodgkin's disease

A small deposit of the mixed-cell variety occupies a portal tract. Reed–Sternberg cells are often inconspicuous in hepatic lesions, but one is present in this deposit (arrow). Extensive involvement of portal tracts with destruction of bile ducts may explain the cholestatic jaundice which may occur in at least a proportion of these cases. These intrahepatic deposits always involve portal tracts. Usually they are of the mixed-cell or nodular sclerosing varieties of the disease. × 117 Hematoxylin and eosin.

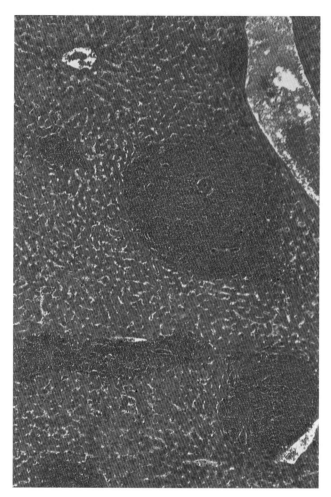

10.81 Lymphosarcoma involving liver.

10.86 Liver in mastocytosis

A toluidine blue preparation which shows several round or spindle-shaped mast cells with purple metachromatic cytoplasm (arrows). This patient had suffered from urticaria pigmentosa for several years before developing signs of a visceral mastocytosis. Liver biopsy is useful in establishing this diagnosis. × 234 Toluidine blue.

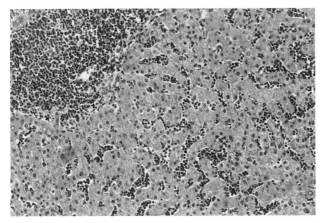

10.82 Liver in leukemia.

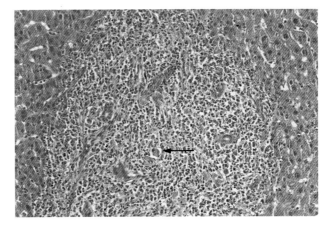

10.85 Liver in Hodgkin's disease.

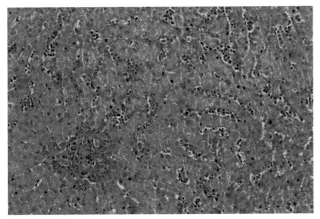

10.83 Liver in leukemia.

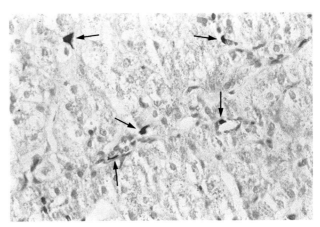

10.86 Liver in mastocytosis.

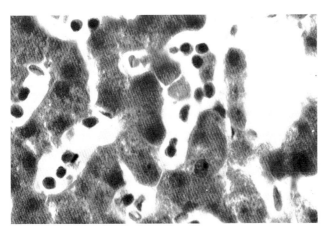

10.84 Liver in leukemia.

CHAPTER 11

Developmental Anomalies

11.1 Solitary (non-parasitic) cyst

On the undersurface of the left lobe of the liver there is a large thin-walled cyst which contained clear serous fluid. These lesions may be unilocular or multilocular and are usually without clinical features unless of very large size.

11.2 Adult polycystic disease

An area of polycystic disease occupies the centre of this liver slice. This is a small part of a greatly enlarged liver about eighty per cent of which consisted only of cysts. The cysts contained thin pale yellow mucinous fluid, and are unusual in this case in possessing also numerous small biliary stones. A larger stone was present in the common bile duct and caused obstructive jaundice.

11.3 Adult polycystic disease

The cysts are for the most part thin-walled, consisting of fibrous connective tissue and lined by cuboidal or low columnar epithelium. × 20 Hematoxylin and eosin.

11.4 Adult polycystic disease

A higher magnification of the specimen shown in **11.3**. In this area the cyst wall is relatively thick and includes a number of dilated vascular channels and small bile ductules. × 75 Hematoxylin and eosin.

11.5 Childhood polycystic disease

This infant's liver showed little gross abnormality but was diffusely involved by proliferation of bile ductular channels, many of which show cystic dilatation. These channels are lined by cuboidal epithelium which formed polypoid projections into a few larger cystic spaces (not shown here). The amount of fibrous stroma is variable and may be minimal around some lesions. Within the liver parenchyma are small dark foci of hematopoiesis, a normal feature for a patient of this age. This condition is different from the adult form of polycystic disease in being autosomal recessive (the adult disease is autosomal dominant), and having a more constant association with renal developmental anomalies. × 71 Hematoxylin and eosin.

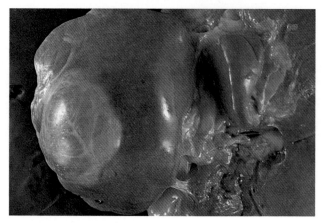

11.1 Solitary (non-parasitic) cyst.

11.6 von Meyenburg complex

This consists of small collections of dilated bile ductular channels set in a fibrous stroma and is found not infrequently. It has been regarded as a minor form of adult polycystic disease. The surrounding liver is normal. × 47 Hematoxylin and eosin.

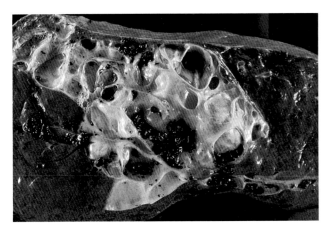

11.2 Adult polycystic disease.

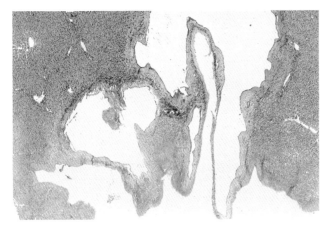

11.3 Adult polycystic disease.

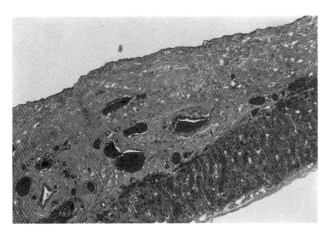

11.4 Adult polycystic disease.

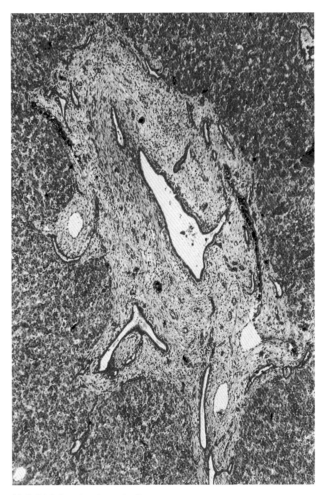

11.5 Childhood polycystic disease.

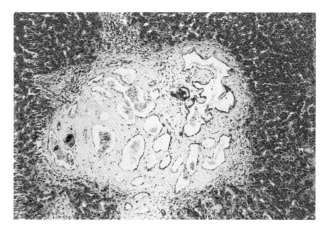

11.6 von Meyenburg complex.

11.7 Congenital hepatic fibrosis

The cut surface of the liver shows numerous small stellate foci of fibrosis, some connected by thin septa. There are no cysts and no hyperplastic nodules indicative of cirrhosis.

11.8 Congenital hepatic fibrosis

The liver is intersected by bands of fibrous connective tissue, of variable shapes and thicknesses, which contain numerous bile ductular structures. The smaller ductules tend to be aggregated at the margins of the fibrous lesions and a few are dilated and contain inspissated bile (arrow). Smaller lesions as seen on the right consist mainly of ductules. The intervening liver parenchyma shows no nodular regeneration. Some of these lesions also contain abnormal vascular channels which may be related to the severe portal hypertension which frequently accompanies this disease. × 47 Van Gieson's stain and hematoxylin.

11.9 Congenital hepatic fibrosis

A broad band of red fibrous tissue is lined with bile ductules which consist of small deeply staining cuboidal epithelium. Cholestasis is present (bottom right). Some ductules (top left) appear unrelated to fibrous tissue. × 117 Van Gieson's stain and hematoxylin.

11.10 Congenital hepatic fibrosis: cholangitis

Individuals with this condition are prone to biliary infection especially after surgical operations for the relief of portal hypertension. Numerous acute inflammatory cells fill most of the bile ductules in this field, and a little bile pigment is present also (arrows). × 88 Hematoxylin and eosin.

11.11 Congenital hepatic fibrosis: mild case

Congenital hepatic fibrosis is discovered generally in children and young adults, but in older patients with portal hypertension, histological examination of the liver occasionally shows minor degrees of the disease, as in this case. Here the lesions consist mostly of small groups of bile ductules while fibrosis is relatively inconspicuous. × 47 Hematoxylin and eosin.

11.12 Cystic dilatation of intrahepatic bile ducts (Caroli's disease)

A grossly dilated intrahepatic bile duct has a thick fibrous wall and contains inspissated bile pigment. These cystic lesions are in continuity with normal bile ducts. They may involve segments of ducts within and outwith the liver. × 32 Hematoxylin and eosin.

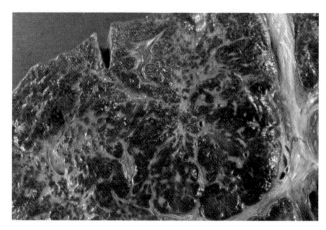

11.7 Congenital hepatic fibrosis.

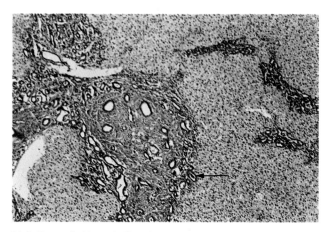

11.8 Congenital hepatic fibrosis.

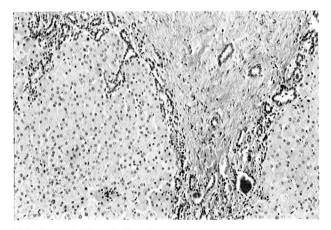

11.9 Congenital hepatic fibrosis.

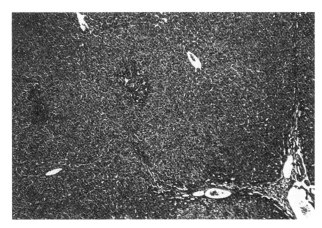

11.11 Congenital hepatic fibrosis: mild case.

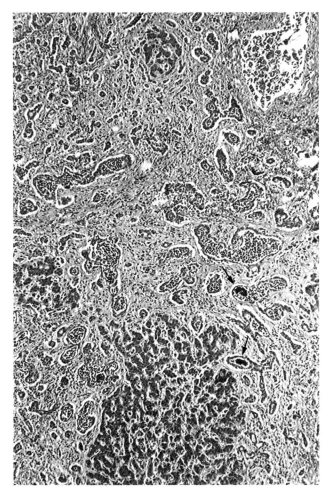

11.10 Congenital hepatic fibrosis: cholangitis.

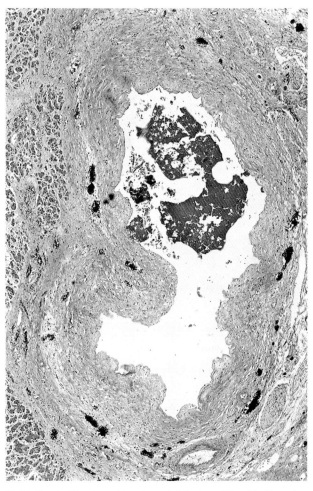

11.12 Cystic dilatation of intrahepatic bile ducts (Caroli's disease).

11.13 Intrahepatic biliary atresia

This is a section of liver obtained post mortem from a child aged eighteen months who suffered from cholestatic jaundice. There is extensive fibrosis of two portal tracts which contain no interlobular bile ducts although there is ductular proliferation at their margins. Cholestasis also is evident. The entire liver was similarly affected. Progression to cirrhosis is very unusual in such cases. This is probably not a single disease entity. Intrahepatic biliary damage and portal fibrosis may be a consequence of some acquired viral infection of liver or cholangitis, secondary to extrahepatic biliary atresia. It may be found also in association with certain recognizable chromosomal defects such as trisomy 17-18 and Down's syndrome or with disorders of bile metabolism. It may be an important component of one genetically determined syndrome which also includes developmental anomalies of the vertebral column, pulmonary stenosis and growth retardation. × 45 Hematoxylin and eosin.

11.14 Intrahepatic gallbladder

The cystic structure with corrugated wall on the left is part of the gallbladder which was situated entirely within the liver. This was an incidental finding at post-mortem examination. The condition is probably unimportant unless in patients requiring cholecystectomy.

11.15 Hepatic herniation through a defect in the diaphragm

Dissection of the thorax and abdomen of this still-born full-term infant shows part of the liver in the right thoracic cavity with displacement of the heart (arrow) to the patient's left. The incompletely formed right dome of diaphragm lies within a fissure which separates thoracic from abdominal portions of the liver. This defect is not incompatible with survival and surgical repair may be possible, but this infant had other serious developmental anomalies. It is a consequence of failure in development of part of the diaphragm. The presence of liver in the thorax may be mistaken clinically for a thoracic neoplasm.

11.16 Partial nodular transformation of liver

Several indistinct pale nodules are seen within the substance of the liver; these are areas of liver parenchymal hyperplasia and there is no accompanying fibrosis. The nodules were larger and more numerous in the region of the porta hepatis and a cause of severe portal hypertension which led to the death of this patient at the age of twenty-three years. These lesions may be confined to the deeper parts of the liver and be missed in routine needle aspiration specimens. The pathogenesis of this condition is unclear and it is suggested that certain cases may be the result rather than the cause of portal venous thrombosis which may co-exist. This patient had suffered from serious portal hypertension since early childhood and cavernomatous transformation of the portal vein (3.16) was discovered at autopsy.

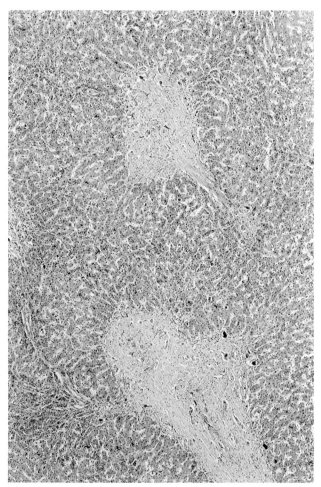

11.13 Intrahepatic biliary atresia.

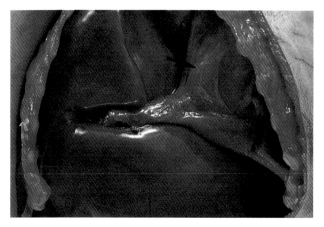

11.15 Hepatic herniation through a defect in the diaphragm.

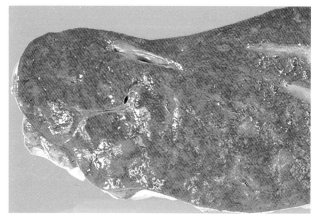

11.16 Partial nodular transformation of liver.

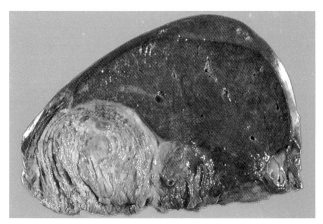

11.14 Intrahepatic gallbladder.

CHAPTER 12

Effects on Other Organs and Tissues

The following conditions arise frequently but not exclusively as complications of established liver disease. Other conditions which have only a coincidental association, e.g. alcoholic cardiomyopathy, are excluded.

12.1 Congestive splenomegaly in portal hypertension

This shows the cut surface of a firm congested spleen which weighed 450 gm. The patient had portal hypertension due to hepatic cirrhosis. The splenic capsule is thickened and there is a fibrous adhesion on its upper surface (right). The cut surface appears fibrotic as well as congested although the markings are partly obscured in a small area of early autolysis (centre left). There are four small pale subcapsular infarcts and a fifth infarct within the substance of the organ (arrow). These fibrotic and vascular changes are consequences of chronic portal hypertension, and lesser degrees may be seen in systemic venous congestion. Some patients with congestive splenomegaly have splenic anemia but this complication is not associated with any special structural changes in the organ.

12.2 Congestive splenomegaly

The red pulp shows diffuse thickening of sinusoidal walls. Some sinusoids appear to be empty despite overall congestion of the spleen. Two Malpighian bodies are present in this field but in other parts of the organ many had undergone atrophy or fibrosis. × 35 Hematoxylin and eosin.

12.3 Congestive splenomegaly: Gandy–Gamna body

There is much dark hemosiderin pigment in this large nodule adjacent to a splenic vein and within a thickened fibrous trabecula. This is a Gandy–Gamna body. These bodies may be seen on naked-eye examination of the cut surface of the spleen as small brown foci with pale centres. × 47 Hematoxylin and eosin.

12.4 Congestive splenomegaly: Gandy–Gamna body

The same lesion as illustrated in **12.3** treated by Perls' method to demonstrate the Prussian blue reaction of iron-containing pigment within the siderotic nodule. × 36 Perls' method and neutral red.

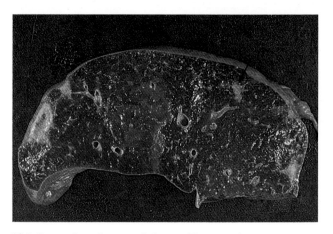

12.1 Congestive splenomegaly in portal hypertension.

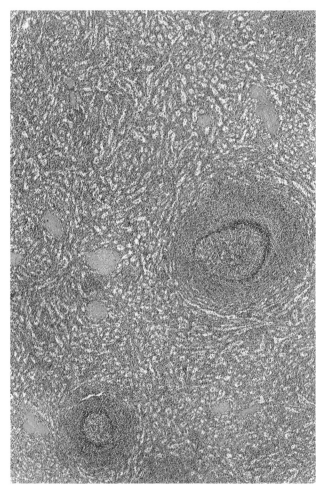

12.2 Congestive splenomegaly.

158

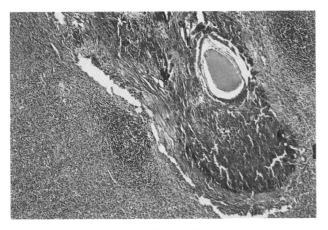

12.3 Congestive splenomegaly: Gandy–Gamna body.

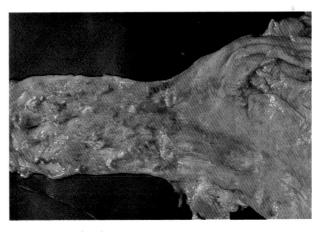

12.5 Esophageal varices.

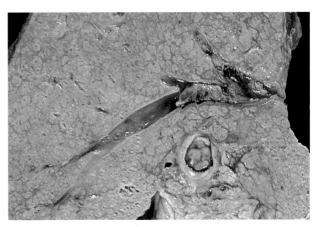

12.6 Portal venous thrombosis.

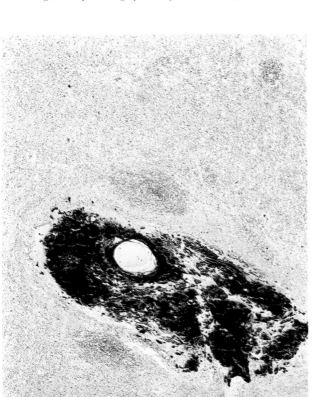

12.4 Congestive splenomegaly: Gandy–Gamna body.

12.5 Esophageal varices

There is striking varicosity of the submucous veins in the wall of the lower end of the esophagus and cardiac end of stomach. This patient suffered from hepatic cirrhosis with portal hypertension. Serious hemorrhage may arise from mucosal ulceration which involves these vessels.

12.6 Portal venous thrombosis

This is a slice of alcoholic cirrhotic liver which includes the region of the porta hepatis. Pale thrombus is present within several large portal venous channels which has formed as a complication of chronic portal hypertension with atherosclerotic changes in the vessel walls (not visible here). The onset of thrombosis may be indicated by increased severity of ascites.

159

12.7 Testicular atrophy

Impotence is a common complication of chronic liver disease in males and is accompanied by testicular atrophy. This section of testis from a patient with cirrhosis shows thick-walled tubules with loss of germinal epithelium and absence of interstitial cells. Some of these patients also suffer from gynecomastia. Liver disease is associated with multiple sex hormone abnormalities but the pathogenesis of testicular atrophy is uncertain. × 71 Hematoxylin and eosin.

12.8 Spider nevus

This is a typical example in the skin of forearm. Each lesion consists of dilated dermal vessels radiating from a central arteriole. Spider nevi occur in the upper part of the body. Palmar erythema may also be present. Both types of lesion have been attributed to failure of diseased liver to inactivate estrogens but the real pathogenesis is unknown.

12.9 Cirrhotic glomerulonephritis

The two glomeruli in this field show some evidence of cellular proliferation with increase in mesangium. Blood cells are inconspicuous and there is no membranous thickening. Despite the resemblance to proliferative glomerulonephritis there is usually no history of streptococcal infection or clinical evidence of renal dysfunction and hypertension. The association with cirrhosis is unclear but glomerulonephritis may be an extrahepatic manifestation of hepatitis B infection. × 234 Hematoxylin and eosin.

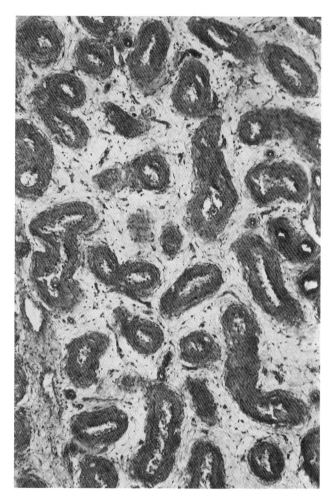

12.7 Testicular atrophy.

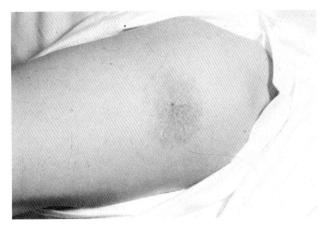

12.8 Spider nevus.

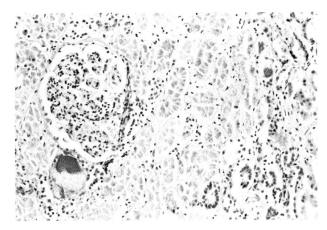

12.10 Hepato-renal syndrome.

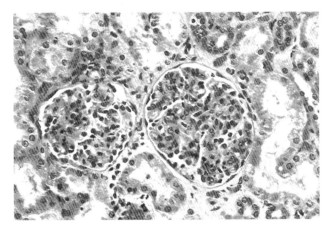

12.9 Cirrhotic glomerulonephritis.

12.10 Hepato-renal syndrome

This post-mortem kidney from a case of hepato-renal syndrome shows tubular necrosis with bile-stained casts. The syndrome is usually attributed to renal damage from shock in a patient who happens to be jaundiced, and it would appear that severe cholestatic jaundice confers unusual susceptibility to the damaging effects of acute circulatory failure on the kidney. Accordingly, the hepato-renal syndrome is a recognized complication of surgical treatment of severe biliary disease. ×117 Hematoxylin and eosin.

12.11 Peripheral blood: macrocytosis

Compared with normal erythrocytes the cells in this blood film are abnormally thin and have an increased diameter. Macrocytosis is a common finding in patients with liver disease from various causes. Apparently it is a consequence of non-specific hepatic parenchymal damage and is unrelated to deficiency of vitamin B12 or folate. Anemia may occur in liver disease for a variety of reasons such as alimentary bleeding, hypersplenism, folate deficiency and excessive hemolysis. × 468 Leishman's stain.

12.12 Peripheral blood: target cells

At least three erythrocytes (arrows) in this field are typical target cells. These cells may be found in patients with liver disease, especially when there is cholestatic jaundice. The pathogenesis is uncertain but is probably related to an increase in cell membrane cholesterol which occurs as a result of elevated circulating bile salts. Target cells may also occur in other blood diseases such as iron deficiency anemia and thalassemia. × 670 Leishman's stain.

12.13 Peripheral blood: stomatocytosis

Each of several red cells (arrows) possesses a pale oval area ('keyhole abnormality'). This abnormality is due to a dimple on one side of the cell and is characteristic of the stomatocyte. Stomatocytosis may occur in various types of chronic liver disease and also in certain hemolytic disorders. × 536 Leishman's stain.

12.14 Peripheral blood: acanthocytosis

This blood film contains numerous acanthocytes or 'spur cells' which are red cells with multiple spicules projecting from their surfaces. These cells have a shortened survival time and the patient may suffer from hemolytic anemia. Acanthocytosis is found in liver disease from various causes. × 693 Leishman's stain.

12.15 Hepatic encephalopathy

Several Alzheimer type II astrocytes are present in this field, which is taken from the cerebellum of a fatal case of hepatic failure. The abnormal cells (arrows) have enlarged and irregularly shaped nuclei with prominent nuclear membrane and inconspicuous cytoplasm. With appropriate staining glycogen can be demonstrated within the nuclei. Proliferation and degeneration of these protoplasmic astrocytes may be related to disturbed ammonia metabolism with accumulation of glutamine in the brain which occurs in hepatic failure. Neuronal damage and demyelination may occur also but are not specific. × 300 Hematoxylin and eosin.

12.16 Kernicterus

This section through an infant's brain shows bile staining of basal ganglia in the centre of the field. This child suffered from neonatal hepatitis and died within a few days of birth. Kernicterus is a serious complication of unconjugated hyperbilirubinemia which need not be due to a primary liver disease; indeed, many are due to hemolytic disease of newborn and hyperbilirubinemia of prematurity. Bile staining of brain is associated with loss of ganglion cells and gliosis, and in those cases who survive there are neurological disorders which usually include muscle spasticity or hypotonia and deafness.

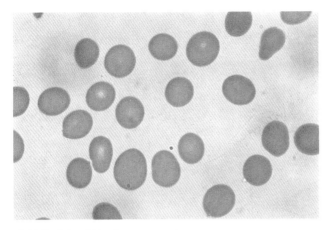

12.11 Peripheral blood: macrocytosis.

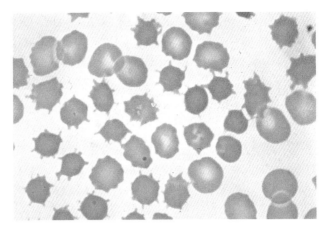

12.14 Peripheral blood: acanthocytosis.

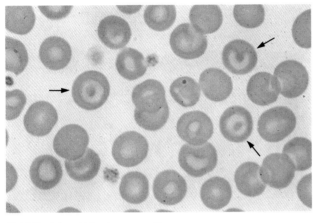

12.12 Peripheral blood: target cells.

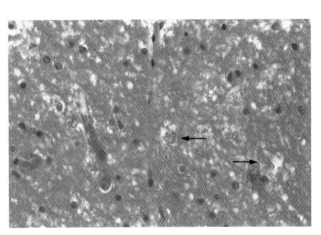

12.15 Hepatic encephalopathy.

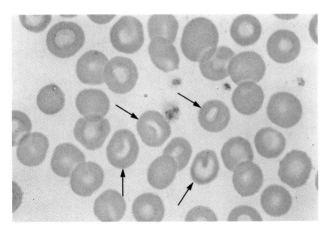

12.13 Peripheral blood: stomatocytosis.

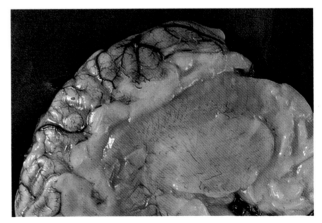

12.16 Kernicterus.

Bibliography

A bibliography prepared for all the conditions illustrated or mentioned in the text would result in a very long list of references inappropriate to an atlas of pathology. This information may be obtained readily in the following books devoted to liver disease:

Liver Disease in General

Schiff L ed. Diseases of the Liver. Philadelphia: J B Lippincott, 4th edition 1975

Sherlock S. Disease of the Liver and Biliary system. Oxford: Blackwell Scientific Publications, 6th edition 1981

Wright R, Alberti K G M M, Karran S and Millward-Sadler G H eds. Liver and Biliary Disease. Philadelphia: W B Saunders, 1979

Liver Pathology

MacSween R N M, Anthony P P and Scheuer P J eds. Pathology of the Liver. Edinburgh: Churchill Livingstone, 1979

Liver Biopsy

Patrick R S and McGee J O'D. Biopsy Pathology of the Liver. London: Chapman and Hall, 1980

Poulsen H and Christoffersen P. Atlas of Liver Biopsies. Copenhagen: Munksgaard, 1979

Scheuer P J. Liver Biopsy Interpretation. London: Bailliere Tindall, 3rd edition 1980

Additional accounts of certain important aspects of liver pathology may be found in the following books and review articles:

Normal liver structure and function

Jones A L and Schmucker D L. Current concepts of liver structure as related to function. Gastroenterology 1977; 73, 833–851

Rappaport A M. The microcirculatory acinar concept of normal and pathological hepatic structure. Beitr Pathol 1976; 157, 215–243

Wisse E and Knook D L eds. Kupffer Cells and other Liver Sinusoidal Cells. Amsterdam: Elsevier, 1977

Cholestasis and biliary obstruction

Christoffersen P and Poulsen H. Histological changes in human liver biopsies following extrahepatic biliary obstruction. Acta Pathol Microbiol Scand 1970; Supplement 212: 150–157

Gentilini P, Teodori U, Gorini S and Popper H eds. Intrahepatic cholestasis. New York: Raven Press, 1975

Popper H and Schaffner F. Pathophysiology of cholestasis. Hum Pathol 1970; 1: 1–24

Vascular disorders

Bras G. Aspects of hepatic vascular disease. In Gall E A and Mostofi F K eds. The Liver. International Academy of Pathology Monograph 13, Baltimore: Williams and Wilkins, 1972; 406–430

Toxic and drug-induced injuries

Bianchi L et al. Guidelines for diagnosis of therapeutic drug-induced liver injury in liver biopsies. Lancet 1974; i: 854–857

Maddrey W C and Boitnott J K. Drug-induced chronic liver disease. Gastroenterology 1977; 72: 1348–1353

Sherlock S. Hepatic reactions to drugs. Gut 1979; 20: 634–638

Zimmerman H J. Hepatotoxicity. New York: Appleton-Century-Crofts, 1976

Alcoholic and nutritional diseases

Fisher M M and Rankin J G eds. Alcohol and the Liver, Vol 3. New York: Plenum Press, 1977

Hoyumpa A M, Green H C, Dunn G D and Schenker S. Fatty liver: biochemical and clinical considerations. Am J Digest Dis 1975; 20: 1142–1170

Macsween R N M. Alcoholic liver disease. In Anthony P P and Woolf N eds. Recent Advances in Histopathology 10. Edinburgh: Churchill Livingstone, 1978: 193–212

Peters R L, Gay T and Reynolds T B. Post-jejunoileal-bypass hepatic disease: its similarity to alcoholic liver disease. Am J Clin Pathol 1975; 63: 318–331

Viral hepatitis

Bianchi L et al. Morphological criteria in viral hepatitis: review by an international group. Lancet 1971; i: 333–337

Bianchi L et al. Acute and chronic hepatitis revisited. Lancet 1977; ii: 914–919

Ishak K C. Light microscopic morphology of viral hepatitis. Am J Clin Pathol 1976; 65: 787–827

Krugman S and Gocke D J. Viral Hepatitis. Philadelphia: W B Saunders, 1978

Sherlock S ed. Viral Hepatitis. Clinics in Gastroenterology Vol 9, 1. Philadelphia: W B Saunders, 1980

The Committee on Viral Hepatitis of the Assembly of Life Sciences, National Research Council, USA. Proceedings of a symposium on viral hepatitis. Am J Med Sci 1975; 270: 1–412

Chronic hepatitis and hepatic fibrosis

Anthony P P, Ishak K G, Nayk N C, Poulsen H E, Scheuer P J and Sobin L H. The morphology of cirrhosis: definition, nomenclature and classification. Bull WHO 1977; 55: 521–540

Eddlestone A L W E, Weber J C P and Williams R. Immune reactions in liver disease. Philadelphia: Lippincott, 1979

Gerlach U, Pott G, Rauterberg E W and Voss P eds. Connective tissue of the normal and fibrotic human liver: present state of biochemistry, clinical evaluation and treatment. International Symposium. Munster, 1980. Stuttgart: Georg Thieme Verlag, 1982

McGee J O'D and Fallon A. Hepatic cirrhosis—a collagen formative disease? J Clin Pathol 1978; 31, Supplement 12: 150–157

Popper H. Pathological aspects of cirrhosis: a review. Am J Pathol 1977; 87: 227–264

Schaffner F. Primary Biliary Cirrhosis. Clinics in Gastroenterology Vol 4, 1975; 351–366

Non-viral infections

Edington G M and Gilles H M. Pathology in the Tropics. London: Arnold, 2nd edition 1976

Marcial-Rojas R A. Parasitic disease of the liver. In Gall E A and Mostofi F K eds. The Liver. International Academy of Pathology Monograph 1973; 13: 431–465

Metabolic disorders

Alagille D and Odievre M. Liver and Biliary Tract Disease in Children. New York: John Wiley, 1979

Bondy P K and Rosenberg L E eds. Metabolic control and disease. Philadelphia: W B Saunders, 8th edition 1980

Ishak K G, Edwards R H and Scheuer P J. Pathology of inborn errors of metabolism. In Anthony P P and Woolf N eds. Recent Advances in Histopathology. Edinburgh: Churchill Livingstone, 1978; 10: 91–137

Johannessen J V ed. Electron microscopy in human medicine: Vol 8, The liver, gall-bladder and bile-ducts. New York: McGraw-Hill, 1978; 20–79

Mowat A P. Liver Disorders in Childhood. London: Butterworth, 1979

Powell L W and Kerr J F R. The pathology of the liver in haemochromatosis. In Iochim H L ed. Pathobiology Annual. New York: Appleton-Century-Crofts, 1975; 317–337

Tumours of liver

Cameron H M, Linsell D A and Warwick G P eds. Liver Cell Cancer. Amsterdam: Elsevier, 1976

Gibson J B et al. Histological typing of tumours of the liver, biliary tract and pancreas. International histological classification of tumours 20. Geneva: WHO, 1978

Okuda K and Peters R L eds. Hepatocellular Carcinoma. New York: John Wiley, 1976

Remnar H, Bolt H M, Bannesch P and Popper H. Primary liver tumours. Falk Symposium 25. Lancaster: MTP Press, 1977

Index

Principal references are printed in bold type